THINKING THROUGH RESISTANCE

Acts of public defiance towards biomedical public health policies have occurred throughout modern history, from resistance to early smallpox vaccines in 19th-century Britain and America to more recent intransigence to efforts to contain the Ebola outbreak in Central and West Africa.

Thinking Through Resistance examines a diverse range of case studies of opposition to biomedical public health policies – from resistance to HPV vaccinations in Texas to disputes over HIV prevention research in Malawi – to assess the root causes of opposition. It is argued that far from being based on ignorance, resistance instead serves as a form of advocacy, calling for improvements in basic health-care delivery alongside expanded access to infrastructure and basic social services. Building on this argument, the authors set out an alternative to the current technocratic approach to global public health, extending beyond greater distribution of medical technologies to build on the perspectives of a political economy of health.

With contributions from medical anthropologists, sociologists, and public health experts, *Thinking Through Resistance* makes important reading for researchers, students, and practitioners in the fields of public health, medical anthropology, and public policy.

Nicola Bulled is a medical anthropologist at Worcester Polytechnic Institute, USA. Her research explores the relationships between society and biomedical technologies for improved global health delivery.

Advances in Critical Medical Anthropology
Series Editors: Merrill Singer and Pamela Erickson

This book series advances our understanding of the complex and rapidly changing landscape of health, disease, and treatment around the world with original and innovative books in the spirit of critical medical anthropology that exemplify and extend its theoretical and empirical dimensions. Books in the series address topics across the broad range of subjects addressed by medical anthropologists and other scholars and practitioners working at the intersections of social science and medicine.

Titles in series
The Healthy Ancestor: Embodied Inequality and the Revitalization of Native Hawaiian Health, Juliet McMullin

Drug Effects: Khat in Biocultural and Socioeconomic Perspective, Lisa L. Gezon

Syndemic Suffering: Social Distress, Depression, and Diabetes among Mexican Immigrant Women, Emily Mendenhall

Health Policy in Crisis: Access to Abortion in the Context of Austerity, Bayla Ostrach

Thinking through Resistance: Case Studies of Opposition to Contemporary Global Health Practices, Nicola Bulled

THINKING THROUGH RESISTANCE

A Study of Public Oppositions to Contemporary Global Health Practice

Edited by Nicola Bulled

Routledge
Taylor & Francis Group
NEW YORK AND LONDON

First published 2017
by Routledge
711 Third Avenue, New York, NY 10017

and by Routledge
2 Park Square, Milton Park, Abingdon, Oxon, OX14 4RN

Routledge is an imprint of the Taylor & Francis Group, an informa business

British Library Cataloguing in Publication Data
A catalogue record for this book is available from the British Library

Library of Congress Cataloging in Publication Data
A catalog record for this book has been requested

ISBN: 978-1-62958-334-1 (hbk)
ISBN: 978-1-62958-335-8 (pbk)
ISBN: 978-1-315-20968-5 (ebk)

Typeset in Bembo
by diacriTech, Chennai

TABLE OF CONTENTS

LIST OF CONTRIBUTORS

Judith Barker is a Professor with the Department of Anthropology, History, and Social Medicine at the University of California, San Francisco. Her research has encompassed a variety of qualitative approaches as well as mixed methods studies examining gender, age, and ethnic differences in understanding and management of a variety of illnesses. A sociocultural anthropologist by training, Barker's prevention-oriented, community-based research has examined the beliefs, perceptions, and experiences of health/illness and health care to laypeople, their use of informal support services and resources, and their interface with the formal health-care system. Focusing on patients' understanding of their illness and their day-to-day management strategies, she has focused on health disparities in vulnerable populations, examining structural, familial, and individual contexts that give rise to health disparities.

Ambar Basu is an Associate Professor and Director of Graduate Studies at the University of South Florida, Department of Health Communication, Culture, Postcolonial and Subaltern Studies. His research focuses on health communication, culture, and marginalization. Specifically, Dr. Basu's research positions culture and health communication within the transformational politics of broader theoretical and methodological frameworks such as postcolonial and subaltern studies and critical ethnography. He is currently Senior Editor of the journal *Health Communication*. His recent and ongoing projects look at HIV/AIDS communication practices in sex worker communities and among minority men who have sex with men, philanthropy in health, and issues in global health and medicine. Embedded within his ethnographic research and postcolonial studies, Dr. Basu employs reflexivity as a methodology, questioning his own self, his politics, and his privilege, reflecting inward and deconstructing the lens(es) he uses to engage in knowledge creation.

Nicola Bulled is a teaching professor with Worcester Polytechnic Institute's Interdisciplinary and Global Studies Division. As a medical anthropologist, her research focuses on the biopolitics of global infectious disease prevention and management efforts. She has worked with disadvantaged and vulnerable populations in the U.S., Lesotho, and South Africa. She has also worked on public health programming projects with the Colorado Department of Public Health and Environment, Boston Medical Center, Boston University, Institute for Community Health in Cambridge, Boston Public Health Commission, Massachusetts State Laboratory Institute, and the Centers for Disease Control. She completed a two-year NIH/Fogarty Foundation–funded postdoctoral fellowship with the University of Virginia's Center for Global Health, where she engaged in two primary projects. The first examined the intersections of citizenship, emotional distress, and water insecurity. The second explored the relationship between medical plurality and HIV care outcomes. Her dissertation work funded by the Fulbright Foundation examined the politics of biomedical HIV knowledge among youth in urban and rural areas of Lesotho and formed the basis of her book *Prescribing HIV Prevention: Brining Culture into Global Health Communication* published by Left Coast Press in 2015. She is particularly keen on applying her research to raise awareness of the agency of local populations and the need to include local stakeholders at national and community levels when developing health-related interventions.

Edward Chigwedere is an independent public health and bioethics researcher based in Malawi. Over the past 18 years, he has worked in a number of Southern African Development Committee (SADC) countries. His areas of research interest include HIV/AIDS; maternal, newborn, and child health; family planning; sexual and reproductive health; and water and sanitation.

Christopher J. Colvin is the Head of the Division of Social and Behavioral Sciences at the University of Cape Town in South Africa. He is also a visiting faculty member at the University of Virginia's Department of Public Health Sciences. His research interests include HIV and masculinity, health activism and community health governance, trauma, subjectivity and narrative, and the interface between communities and health systems in the context of HIV/AIDS, TB, and maternal and child health.

Mohan J. Dutta is Provost's Chair Professor and Head of the Department of Communications and New Media at the National University of Singapore (NUS), Adjunct Professor at the Interactive Digital Media Institute (IDMI) at NUS, and Courtesy Professor of Communication at Purdue University. At NUS, he is the Founding Director of the Center for Culture-Centered Approach to Research and Evaluation (CARE), directing research on culturally-centered, community-based projects of social change. He teaches and conducts research in international health communication, critical cultural theory, poverty in healthcare, health activism in globalization politics, indigenous cosmologies of health, subaltern studies and dialogue, and public policy and participatory social change. At the core of his research agenda is the activist emphasis on provincializing Eurocentric knowledge structures and de-centering hegemonic knowledge constructions through subaltern participation. Dr. Dutta has published over 170 journal articles and book chapters. He has authored, co-authored, and co-edited seven books. His recent book *Neoliberal Health Organizing*, published by Left Coast Press, explores the ways in which meanings of health circulating within dominant political, economic, and social structures of global organizing threaten human health and well-being. Currently, he serves as Editor of the *Critical Cultural Studies in Global Health Communication* book series with Left Coast Press/Routledge and sits on the editorial board of seven journals.

Morenike Oluwatoyin Folayan is an Associate Professor at Obafemi Awolowo University in Nigeria. She has worked extensively in the field of biomedical HIV prevention research and advocates for community engagement in research in general and HIV biomedical research and development specifically. She is the author of over 120 peer-reviewed articles. She is currently working on co-authoring a book manuscript with Kristin Peterson, *The Trials and Tribulations of Clinical Research in Africa*. Her work on HIV prevention has focused on addressing the needs of key target populations which are most at risk of HIV infection yet which are often the least addressed in HIV policy planning.

Samantha D. Gottlieb has a master's in health science from Bloomberg School of Public Health and a Ph.D. in Anthropology from Johns Hopkins University. She has worked in the biomedical private sector, with public health departments, and is currently a lecturer at California State University, East Bay. Her research looks at public acceptance and utilization of new medical technologies.

Edward C. Green is a research professor at George Washington University. He was a Senior Research Scientist at the Harvard School of Public Health and served as director of the AIDS Prevention Research Project at the Harvard Center for Population and Development Studies. He has also been affiliated with Johns Hopkins University. He was appointed to serve as a member of the Presidential Advisory Council on HIV/AIDS (2003–2007), served on the Office of AIDS Research Advisory Council for the National Institutes of Health (2003–2006), and serves on the board of AIDS.org. He has worked for over 30 years in international development, much of it in AIDS and sexually transmitted diseases, primarily in Africa, but also in Asia, Latin America, the Caribbean, the Middle East, and Eastern Europe. He has published numerous books, most recently *AIDS, Behavior, and Culture* (with Allison Ruark) and *Broken Promises: How the AIDS Establishment Has Betrayed the Developing World*. He is currently working on archiving his years of fieldwork for the Smithsonian's National Anthropology Archives.

Sarah Horton is a medical anthropologist whose research interests include migration and health – the global linkages between health-care systems, farm worker, and cross-border health. She was research faculty at the University of California, San Francisco, from 2005 until 2007, where she served as lead ethnographer on a project funded by the National Institute of Dental and Craniofacial Research that examined the causes of oral health disparities for Latino farm-worker children in California's Central Valley. Dr. Horton's research in the Central Valley examined the dietary, environmental, and cultural factors that contributed to the high rates of oral disease among Latino farm-worker children. Placing immigrant children's oral health disparities in a transnational framework, she examined how Latino immigrant parents' own experiences with oral health in their countries of origin shaped their caregiving practices. She also examined the role of dental Medicaid policy in contributing to farm-worker children's untreated oral disease and in permanently altering their physiognomies in ways that marked them as "second-class citizens."

Alex M. Nading is a lecturer in Social Anthropology at the University of Edinburgh. As a medical and environmental anthropologist, Dr. Nading studies the entanglement of human and non-human lives. He has conducted ethnographic work in Nicaragua since 2006, exploring dengue mosquitoes, dengue viruses, and microbiota. From this, he published his book *Mosquito Trails: Ecology, Health, and the Politics of Entanglement* with the University of California Press in 2014. At present, he is involved in two research projects. The first examines the place of genetically engineered organisms in global health, with a focus on efforts to control the mosquito-borne virus that causes dengue fever. The second draws from his work in Nicaragua as he examines how the global fight against antimicrobial resistance takes hold in the global South.

Evaristo Nthete is a Diagnostic Radiographer and is currently working as a Radiography Lecturer at Malawi College of Health Sciences. He has worked in different hospitals for 13 years and has taught Radiography and Health Research for 15 years. His research areas of interest include HIV and AIDS as well as breast and chest imaging.

Kristin Peterson is an associate professor at the University of California, Irvine. Her research and writing are concerned with theories of capital and property; "popular" economies, trade, and markets; health, science, and medicine studies; and postcolonial theory. Her first book, *Speculative Markets: Drug Circuits and Derivative Life in Nigeria*, was published in 2014 with Duke University Press. Drawing on the stories and lives of industry executives, pharmaceutical market traders, industry and academic pharmacists, drug marketers, narcotics traders, and regulatory officials, she describes the making of drug chemistries and market dynamics in the aftermath of 1980s liberalization. In tying market actors to both local and transcontinental economic strategies, the book resituates how we think about market-making and non-equilibrium theories of neoliberalism in the postcolony and beyond. With

Morenike Folayan Ukpong, she is writing a second book, *The Trials and Tribulations of Clinical Research in Africa. The* focus of this work is on pre-exposure prophylaxis (PrEP) HIV prevention technologies that were designed and funded by U.S. federal government programs, international HIV prevention research consortiums, and international social marketing firms. The authors examine African debates on ethics and clinical research that interface with market logics and extensive trial failure.

Matthew Puffer is a Catherine of Siena Fellow at Villanova University. His research explores competing normative visions of the human person, especially rival versions of the imago dei and human dignity and their implications for issues in biomedical, economic, environmental, and war and peace ethics. He recently co-edited a four-volume collection, *Comparative Religious Ethics: The Major Works*, and has published on the ethics of war, lying, and responsible action in *Modern Theology*, the *International Journal of Systematic Theology*, and edited volumes.

Steven Robins is a Professor in the Department of Sociology and Social Anthropology at the University of Stellenbosch. He has published on a wide range of topics, including the politics of land, 'development,' and identity in Zimbabwe and South Africa; the Truth & Reconciliation Commission (TRC); urban studies; and most recently on citizenship and governance. His book *From Revolution to Rights in South Africa: Social Movements and Popular Politics* (2008) focuses on globally connected social movements, NGOs, and CBOs that are involved in democratic struggles over access to AIDS treatment, land, and housing. He has edited *Limits to Liberation After Apartheid: Citizenship, Governance and Culture* which is published by David Philip, James Currey, and Ohio University Press (2005). His edited volume (with Nick Shepherd) is entitled *New South African Keywords* (Jacana and Ohio University Press, 2008). He is currently working on issues relating to social movements involved in community-based struggles over access to improved public education, health, and sanitation in informal settlements.

1

INTRODUCTION

Thinking Through Resistance

Nicola Bulled and Matthew Puffer

In 2014, as Central and West Africa faced the worst Ebola outbreak in recorded history, it seemed to many that the world was standing by, hardly noticing. Even when the outside world did notice, little was done to actively care for Africa or the thousands that would die from an unanticipated Ebola epidemic born out of a predictably uncoordinated, underfunded, and misdirected global health response. Media accounts of the epidemic in the U.S. called attention less to the social, systemic, and structural shortcomings than to the sensationalized conflicts including scattered attacks on Ebola outbreak teams that resulted in health workers (both foreign and local) being challenged, driven out of villages, and even killed (Nossiter, 2014). Meanwhile, reporting on the complicated histories of exploitative corruption, which would have shed light on the locals' reactions toward individuals and organizations who had come to help, was slow to surface (Fink, 2014). Instead, such reflection was restricted, as usual, to debates among academics and health experts.

The Ebola crisis in West Africa, officially declared over by the World Health Organization (WHO) in January 2016, brought to the fore many long-standing, even historical, concerns over state-organized public health efforts (Garrett, 2015). Local resistance to organized efforts reflects the tension and potential conflict or competition between two narratives about the roles of individuals and of the state in ensuring the health of the public, particularly when resources are scarce. The emerging local narratives about Ebola in Guinea, identified by Fodei Batty (2014), reveal this twofold dynamic as it exists currently through much of the world. The first, individual-centric narrative blames victims of disease for their "ignorance" and "backwardness," and, in the case of Ebola, for their suspicions of modern medicine. This narrative reflects a new public health paradigm that links the responsibility of health directly to the individual who is expected to make rational decisions based on existing knowledge and available resources (Horton & Barker, 2009). By contrast, the second, state-centric narrative draws attention to the responsibility of the state to put in place policies and programming that protects the public. In Guinea, this latter narrative took the form of "conspiracy theories" to explain why remote regions were affected, as opposed to urban areas where the central government is established, as well as why containment was delayed.

Indeed, a lack of trust in government and suspicion of elected officials serves as a central theme in many accounts of the Ebola epidemic, as noted in the "Ebola in Perspective" collection edited by Moran and Hoffman (2014) for the 'Fieldsites' element of *Cultural Anthropology Online*. The distrust and violence directed at Ebola containment efforts appears often related to issues of state legitimacy (Ammann, 2014; Batty, 2014; Schroven, 2014). For example, in Guinea, Batty points to an historical distrust of "foreign elements" developed during the 1990s, when non-government organizations (NGOs) or UN actions accommodated refugee populations and combatants from neighboring countries' civil wars, at the expense of local communities' well-being. Batty suggests that attacks on health centers and the denial of entry to NGO and government health workers to villages within the very heart of the outbreak was a well-established strategy of self-defense against any foreign element, whether combatant, government representative, or international health organization. Anita Schroven (2014) further suggests that because central government agents are so rarely present in the Guinean countryside, and when they are present they accompany NGO campaigns or police missions, the public has predictably learned to perceive government agents as foreign elements, and thus with some suspicion.

In Liberia, Theresa Amman (2014) recounts a similar state of uncertainty and distrust resulting from limited information, delayed government response, centuries of government corruption, and war. With the advance of Ebola, personal insecurity resulted in fear, denial, anger, and confusion. People were unwilling to bring their sick relatives to care facilities, fearing that their condition would worsen because of starvation or that they would never see them again due to prohibited funeral rites. Even if families chose to seek outside assistance, patients were frequently refused entry into care facilities due to overcrowding, further fueling instability, chaos, and confusion. Political insecurity was fostered by an ineffective state of emergency, the dumping of bodies into community wetlands, the shooting of a 16-year-old, the closing of a newspaper over allegations of spreading false information, unknown financial aid allocation, and uncertainty about how, if, and to whom treatment had been distributed (Ammann, 2014). Lacking trust in public authorities, Liberians responded by placing trust in self, family, neighbors, and local religious institutions, and took such actions as self-quarantining and forming Boy Scouts' awareness campaigns and vigilante groups that expelled or quarantined infected people.

These ethnographic accounts reveal that public resistance to Ebola containment efforts were less about public ignorance or concerns driven by exotic cultural differences, as they were about well-informed cultural norms and narratives learned through long histories of state interventions that were far from beneficent. With this history in view, it is understandable and quite predictable that new public health disruptions were interpreted through lenses informed by longstanding perceptions of state and foreign interventions gone awry, including an ongoing contestation regarding the nature of citizen-state relationships. Examining the motivations behind the disruptions caused by the public to officially organized health efforts provides valuable insights on public health programing and delivery.

Recognizing the importance of examining public reactions to health programs, in 1955, Dr. Benjamin Paul, in collaboration with Walter Miller, published a groundbreaking collection of case studies on the public health programing efforts. When this collection was first published, modern medical anthropology was only just beginning to emerge as a subdiscipline of anthropology and distinct from ethnographic work taking place within the medical field. Paul was regarded as "one of the new group of social scientists who [had] taken the time to become familiar with health problems" (Paul, 1955, p. iv). Despite significant advances in biomedicine and epidemiology, medical practitioners working in community medicine, or public health, increasingly realized that "it [was] not easy to persuade the public to make full use of the health information at hand" (Paul, 1955, p. iii). One result of this self-awareness was that public health experts began calling upon social scientists, like Dr. Paul, to assist in as they described: "remov[ing] the veil before our eyes which keeps us from seeing clearly the people we serve" (Leavell in, Paul, 1955, p. iii). Paul's book solidified the application of social-science theory and methods to the practical ends of medicine and public health. This work, and others like it, provided a catalyst and the activation energy for the emergence of a new subfield – *critical medical anthropology*.

Experienced public health workers wrote the cases presented in Paul's collection, providing honest and vulnerable accounts of both successes and failures. Although they are now more than 60 years old, these cases continue to provide useful insights into the struggles of contemporary public health efforts as they illuminate the complexity of the process of engaging with, involving, and in fact, empowering community. In framing the collection, Paul (1955, p. 2) notes:

> We must reexamine the prevalent assumption that good results automatically carry conviction; dramatic effects in preventing or curing illness are not always self-validating. Facts do not speak for themselves; they are always cross-examined and given meaning in accordance with the assumptions of the examiner. We realize almost at once that the mosquito's image of the world must diverge sharply from our own. We realize less readily that different groups of humans, despite their constitutional similarities, can differ significantly and systematically in their perceptions of the same event.

Data is not self-interpreting but is always the product of, and represented by, the interpretive assumptions and lenses of culturally conditioned and socially located human agents. This is a useful starting place for examining contemporary global public health efforts. Despite the concept of cultural diversity being commonplace in disciplines like anthropology, public health as a discipline continues to struggle to consider approaches that valorize diversity.

Like the essays in Paul and Miller's collection, the social scientists that write the essays in our collection make what we take to be a convincing case for the importance of concepts like 'culture' and 'interpretation.' However, this volume's continuity with its antecedents does not entail redundancy nor does it suggest that the generalizable knowledge pursued amounts to a mere reprise of older collections of studies. Indeed, the discipline of medical anthropology has advanced considerably since the efforts of Paul and his contemporaries. Critical medical anthropology (CMA), a branch of medical anthropology advanced by noted scholars such as Merrill Singer, Paul Farmer, Hans Baer, Ida Susser, and Pamela Erickson, has established that while individual personalities, shared culture, and local ecological relationships influence health, so too do the structures of social relationships. For example, there are interactions between the micro-level experiences of individuals and health, the meso-level of social organization and agentive action, and the macro-level of social structure. A new generation of CMA scholars and practitioners give careful attention to the 'vertical links' that connect social groups to the larger regional, national, and global human society, and to the configuration of social relationships (which are often unequal) that contribute to patterns of human behavior, belief, and attitudes.

In this, CMA calls attention to the ways in which people develop their own individual and collective understandings and responses to illness. At the same time, such beliefs and associated actions are formulated in a world that is not entirely of our own making, a world where access to health care, media, information, productive resources, and valued social status remains unequal. Through these principles, CMA addresses the social origins of illness, including the ways in which poverty, discrimination, industrial pollution, and violence contribute to poor health. Among other things, CMA pays attention to the origins of dominant cultural constructions of 'health,' under what set of historic conditions these constructions arise, and which social classes, genders, or ethnic groups' interests particular health concepts express. In doing so, CMA emphasizes structures of power and inequality in health and health-care systems and highlights that certain health ideas and practices can contribute to and reinforce inequalities.

Health is intertwined with the social, the political, the economic, the moral, and the historic. Recognizing this integral ecology, the present volume brings together cases that highlight sites and moments of disruption to public health efforts. Each case is written by anthropologists or academics of a related discipline, some of whom are also trained and experienced public health practitioners with extensive experience in development work, who offer not only their informed ethnographic perspective, but also a view on how each situation relates to the larger regional and global concerns. In focusing on 'disruption,' which some may view as 'failures,' our intention is not to assign blame, either to individual actors, institutions, or to the public health agenda as a whole, whatever that may be. Rather, we want to highlight, as articulated by Julian Brown, that disruptions made by ordinary men and women, asserting themselves as equal global citizens, "expose the ordinary operations of a disempowering order – and may begin to change it" (2015, p. 6). Again, without moralizing or assigning blame, the phenomena of disrupted public health interventions prove useful sites for interrogating the meaning-making enterprise of the public health community, including doctors, researchers, policy advocates, and participants of various sorts. As such, the aim of this collection is to invoke a new and more critically informed conceptualization of the public health agenda which recognizes that, given the opportunity and resources, individuals and communities can identify both particular public health needs and the best public health measures through which to effectively address them.

A brief history of public health: Practices and principles

Public health, the practice of attempting to improve health and quality of life through the prevention and treatment of disease, has a long history. Primitive populations used ritualistic or customary cleanliness and personal hygiene practices to prevent disease. Scholars often relate these practices to religious beliefs about God, evil, and theodicy, and ancient texts regularly present natural disasters, including disease epidemics, as instances of divine judgment upon the wickedness of humankind (Bellah, 2011; Douglas, 2002 [1966]; Leibniz, 1952; Voltaire, 2005). Religious institutions also served as healing spaces, with ancient Egyptian temples and Greek and Roman shrines, serving as the earliest institutions providing disease treatments and cures (Risse, 1999). Observations of the association between polluted water and foul smelling air led to an understanding of natural causes of disease. During the 5th and 4th centuries BCE, the first scientific theory of disease causation (miasmas theory) was established, formulated in the book *Airs, Water, and Places* thought to be written by Greek physician Hippocrates (Rhodes, 2015). This text offers the first systematic attempt to set forth a causal relationship between disease and the environment. Medical technologies advanced around the world, with ancient Chinese medical doctors developing forms of vaccination against smallpox following an epidemic around 1000 BCE. The inhalation of the dried crusts that formed around smallpox lesions offered some immunity as did the scratching of pus from lesions into the skin of uninfected individuals. By Roman times, hygiene reforms resulted in the standardization of sewage and water systems. Hospitals, houses for dispensing charity and medicines, where diseased and destitute were examined by doctors were recorded in India as early as 400 BCE and much later in Asia Minor in the 370s CE (Fa-hsien & Legge, 1886; Wilken, 2012).

The Middle Ages saw the onset of epidemic diseases including smallpox, plague, leprosy, scabies, tuberculosis, anthrax, trachoma, and Black Death. Primary public health approaches to combating these contagious diseases were to isolate known or suspected cases and persons in close contact. Public officials created a system of sanitary control using observation stations, isolation hospitals, and disinfection procedures. Improvements in sanitation included the development of pure water supplies, garbage and sewage disposal, and food inspection.

While no national health policies developed in Europe before the 18th century, local community-based efforts continued. In 1485, the Republic of Venice established a Permanent Court of supervisors of health, with the intent of preventing the spread of disease epidemics into the territory from abroad (Carbone, 1962; da Mosto, n.d.). Scientific advancements during this period, which included better understandings of anatomy and physiology, observations and classifications of disease, and the compilation of demographic statistics, laid the foundations of modern medicine's germ theory and the public health discipline of epidemiology.

By the 18th century, hospitals were developing throughout Europe, and a basic pattern of improvements in public health emerged (Barry & Carruthers, 2005; Rhodes, 2015). Efforts were made to educate the public on health matters. For example, British physician Sir John Pringle published works that discussed the importance of ventilation in military barracks and the provision of latrines for soldiers (Rhodes, 2015). Pringle also published about jail fever (likely typhus), emphasizing cleanliness and personal hygiene. Similarly, in 1754, James Lind published a treatise on scurvy, which he linked to a lack of dietary vitamin C (Rhodes, 2015).

However, it was not until the mid to late 19th century that many attributes of the modern discipline of public health emerged, largely resulting from the unintended consequences of the globalization of science, commerce, and politics through colonization and the Industrial Revolution. With the onset of the Industrial Revolution, mass migrations into urban areas resulted in cramped and unsanitary living conditions and unsafe working environments. Consequently, cholera pandemics devastated Europe between 1829 and 1851.

In England, local and national movements called for social and infrastructural reforms to prevent disease. Sir Edwin Chadwick's report 'The Sanitary Conditions of the Labouring Population,' published in 1842, sparked legislation aimed at improving living conditions. In 1848, the first Public Health Act was passed (Ashton & Ubido, 1991). Under the Public Health Act, the General Board of Health became the central local authority body in English cities managing the supply of water, sewage, drainage, cleansing, and paving. City governments made further reforms, including latrinization, the building of sewers, regular garbage collection, the provision of clean water, and the draining of standing water. By 1875, Parliament had passed acts to tackle the problem of overcrowded housing. The Infectious Disease (Notification) Act in 1889 mandated the reporting of infectious diseases to the local sanitary authority, who responded by removing patients to hospitals and disinfecting homes and properties (Mooney, 2015). These reforms focused largely on the management of populations through hygiene and sanitation efforts, quarantine, and compliance; the beginnings of what French philosopher, Michel Foucault has called "biopower" (Foucault, 2010).

While attention to the health of populations as a whole, as opposed to merely individuals, became a growing concern in rapidly urbanizing Europe, it was even more of a concern for European imperial projects. Differences in disease susceptibility between indigenous populations and European colonists both aided and jeopardized imperial expansion. Disease was both used as a weapon against indigenous populations (with populations purposefully infected with particular diseases such as smallpox), and as justification for imperialism (with the 'savage' body viewed as frail and requiring colonial rule) (Chaplin, 2001; Jones, 2004). As in Europe, structural changes under colonial management resulted in dramatic shifts in the movement of people and livestock in the colonies that stimulated disease epidemics (Lyons, 1992).

In order to manage health, initially in support of the military and European-born administrators and civilians, and then to ensure the working capacity of the laboring indigenous populations, a bureaucracy of colonial medical enterprises was established. Sites of colonial occupation often served as laboratories for medical strategies, including the treatment of sleeping sickness, malaria, tuberculosis, and cholera. Recent theories of the beginnings of the HIV pandemic speculate that such colonial efforts to manage disease (largely through experimentation) may have been the primer that moved the HIV virus from contained infections in rural African populations to epidemics in urban areas (Pepin, 2011).

Reflecting the efforts taking place in Europe in the 19th and early 20th century, colonial medicine largely focused disease prevention on hygiene and sanitation. Increasingly, the lifestyles of non-Europeans were viewed as 'primitive, unclean, and uncivilized.' In South Africa, the Public Health Act of 1897 allowed for black residents of the city of Cape Town to be forcibly relocated away from the city center as a disease prevention measure (Swanson, 1977). Europeans believed that Africans, whose "moral ideas and social habits [were] widely divergent from those of educated Europeans" (Fassin, 2007, p. 132), would avoid being corrupted by civilization and contaminating Europeans with disease if they remained out of town. In the American-occupied Philippines, the U.S. military similarly took a heavy-handed, racialized approach to public health efforts, razing villages, forcibly administering drugs, imposing quarantines, and seizing and cremating bodies of individuals who had died from cholera (Anderson, 2006).

With the advancements of modern medicine, including vaccines and treatments for infectious diseases, a distinct discipline of 'tropical medicine' developed. Patrick Manson and other clinicians clarified tropical diseases as those associated with specific latitudes and regions, many transmitted by insect vectors and caused by parasitic agents, unique from 'cosmopolitan diseases,' such as tuberculosis, that could be found anywhere (Worboys, 1976). Guided by Manson's principles of tropical medicine, British trained-surgeon working in the Indian Medical Service, Ronald Ross, described the role of the *Anopheles* mosquito in the life cycle of the malaria parasite, for which he won the Nobel Prize in 1902. These new principles closely aligned with the shifting logics of imperial governance. Near the close of the 19th century, British colonies under Joseph Chamberlain, moved toward a 'constructive imperialism' strategy – exploiting vast underdeveloped estates using both native and non-native laborers and British settlers – which required attending to the health needs of entire populations. Approaches of tropical medicine relied less on individual treatments and more on environmental changes, such as *Anopheles* mosquito control to prevent malaria as a means to combat the germs that cause disease. This logic resonated with institutions of colonial medicine as they protected the health of indigenous (and non-indigenous populations) without providing direct curative services to native subjects who were generally dealt with as populations, not individuals.

The establishment of effective administrative mechanisms for the supervision and regulation of public health evolved into a shared global concern in the mid-19th century. Public health action in France was deeply influenced by a spirit of social reform, and as such scientific methods for the identification, treatment, and control of communicable disease served as the primary guide for administrative efforts. In Germany, the establishment of hygiene as an experimental laboratory science in 1865 signaled the entrance of science into the field of public health. Through this, public health policy makers were able to claim that efforts to prevent or control disease found their basis in medical science, rather than primarily guided by concerns of economics and politics. Historical and contemporary public health efforts continue to receive criticism on this matter. For example, following a case study of the Rockefeller Foundation's hookworm campaign in Mexico in the 1920s, Armanda Solorzana argued that undue intrusion of politics and economics in public health efforts results in manipulation of results or the inappropriate allocation of resources in order to promote certain agendas (Birn & Solórzano, 1999). Harsh criticisms of the WHO's response to the West African Ebola epidemic of 2014/2015 similarly suggest that politics and economics play influential, if ethically objectionable, roles in global public health agendas (Garrett, 2015).

It was not until the early 20th century that a more formalized global health bureaucracy began to emerge. Organizations such as the Pan American Sanitary Bureau and the Rockefeller Foundation led efforts to control diseases in the colonies and former colonies and formed the foundations upon which later global health institutions developed. A critical analysis of these organizations argues that they perpetuated the knowledge frameworks that took shape within institutions of colonial medicine (Greene, Basilico, Kim, & Farmer, 2013). Their efforts largely focused on populations rather than individuals, on single diseases rather than overall good health, on one-size-fits-all models that allow for breadth and depth but no local contextualization, on cost-effectiveness, and on science-as-truth.

These bureaucratic approaches greatly influenced today's global health institutionalized strategies (Greene et al., 2013). Following World War II, the WHO was formed to serve as the global health advisory and coordinating body with universal membership and a decentralized approach. While unsuccessful in its global malaria eradication efforts in the 1950s and '60s, the organization solidified its important role in managing global health programming with its successful eradication of smallpox. Much like the strategies of colonial medicine, both malaria and smallpox eradication efforts relied on top-down, disease-specific approaches that, whether successful or not, established no permanent health structures to address other diseases, health, and social conditions. We see this same vertical strategy employed today in global polio eradication efforts that appear to have little of the intended 'spillover effects' in support of local health structures (Closser et al., 2014). This technocratic approach, as re-popularized by new global health stakeholders like Bill Gates, aims to identify particular goals then develop specific, often technology focused solutions that are constantly evaluated and revised to achieve successful outcomes, where needs, solutions, and success are determined by external experts (Easterly, 2013). However, it allows little to no room for community involvement to address unique social and economic factors and to challenge the structures of institutional knowledge that have been shaped by social processes deemed 'scientific.' As institutions are slow to change, this arrangement largely remains the current state of global public health, with restrictions placed on both who is invited to the policy-making table (further articulated by Basu and Mohan in this volume), how the global health agenda is prioritized (as described by Peterson and colleagues), and whose knowledge is valorized (discussed by Bulled and Green).

Public health ethics: Reconciling competing obligations

Public health is an inherently ethical pursuit insofar as it aims to benefit others. Of course, intending to benefit, actually benefitting, and benefitting in a way that is fair toward all parties involved are three quite different things. As the brief history of public health above suggests, and as our chapters reveal in greater detail, the good intention (benevolence) of a public health effort guarantees neither a good outcome (beneficence) for the health of the public, nor that such benefits are shared fairly (distributive justice) or brought about fairly (procedural justice). St. Bernard of Clairvaux suggested that the road to hell is paved with good intentions, and public health, at times, sustains this worry. Benevolent intentions do not suffice for an ethics of public health. Instead, we must attend to other moral considerations that chasten such a naïve view, which might give guidance to morally fraught and difficult process of discerning how best to pursue public health interventions, and whether to do so when confronted with disruption and resistance.

In response to historical evolutions in public health efforts, the field of public health ethics emerged as a critical and explicitly normative interlocutor with social, political, and environmental sciences. As James F. Childress and Ruth Gaare Bernheim (2008) have argued:

> Public health involves not only traditional government action to protect the public from imminent threats but also, and more fundamentally, cooperative behavior and relationships of trust in communities, as well as a far-reaching agenda to address complex social, behavioral, and/or environmental conditions that affect health.... Particularly at the local community level, public health interventions, e.g., those that focus on socioeconomic or behavioral risk factors, tend to be multidimensional, sustained over months or years, and context-dependent.

Sharing CMA's concerns for public health practices that attend to issues of justice – both in terms of fair distribution of health outcomes as well as fair processes for marginalized and vulnerable populations – public health ethics offers a useful grammar and framework for critical reflection on population health as a moral *good*. We begin by noting that the health of the public is both a good in itself, intrinsically, and also a good that facilitates others, instrumentally (e.g., labor and leisure, the arts, flourishing families, meaningful relationships, social projects). Thus the pursuit of public health is an act of *beneficence* – *bene factum* meaning a 'good deed' – all things being equal. And yet, as the long history of public health amply demonstrates, all things are rarely, if ever, equal.

CMA has emphasized that public health efforts never occur in a vacuum but always instead within an intricate web of interconnected goods, both individual and social, global and local, some of which reinforce one another and others of which are in tension or competition. To the extent that the health of a population is a human good, its pursuit is inherently ethical (i.e., having to do with good and evil, right and wrong). But, to the extent that the health of a population is one human good among many, not all of which are attainable in a world of limited resources, its pursuit is also inherently contestable and requires ethical justification. Recognizing that population health is one good among many, and that not every public health intervention is equally justifiable, public health ethics exercises critical reflection upon how the particular good of public health and its pursuit function in relation to the status and pursuit of other goods. More specifically, ethical explorations of public health efforts examine and critique the explicit and implicit moral norms operative in deliberations about which interventions are or are not justifiable and, among those that are justifiable, the reasons that some are more or less justifiable than others.

Some historically important public health tools and practices already mentioned above – including surveillance, screening, quarantine, state-sponsored sanitation, and forcible relocation – may be justifiable in some circumstances but not in others. Additionally, the specific ways in which these and other processes are utilized and implemented within public health interventions greatly influence our judgments regarding their ethical justification. The practices and processes of reason-giving, as well as the actual ethical reasons themselves that are exchanged between affected community members and public health officials, collectively evidence that the relevant moral considerations extend beyond the norm of beneficence, even if it does play a particularly foundational role. Available public health tools and practices, the reasons offered for their justification, and the processes by which stakeholders participate in determining and implementing interventions all factor into ethical assessments of the justifiability of public health interventions.

Given our focus on *resistance* to public health interventions, the case studies explored in this volume highlight several different ethical tensions that can arise as local community members and public health officials navigate competing interests within structural inequalities and evolving power dynamics. Quite often, and in diverse ways, ethical tensions can manifest as a conflict between beneficence (e.g., the aims of public health practitioners) and the respect due to persons (e.g., the expressed preferences and way of life of local populations). This particular conflict of moral norms typically arises when public health interventions are at odds with moral norms regarding privacy, confidentiality, liberty, or private property. Such was the case with the Ebola crisis of 2015. In extreme situations for example, an Ebola epidemic or a SARS outbreak where quarantine is part of the response, otherwise binding norms involving the protection of these goods might justifiably be overridden. Likewise, ethical tensions often take the form of a conflict between social utility (e.g., good outcomes for overall population health) and justice (e.g., a fair distribution of the benefits and burdens in public health interventions, including among the most vulnerable and marginalized). The conflict between beneficence and respect for persons is practically baked into the phenomenon of resistance to public health interventions, and the conflict between social utility and justice is a common feature where power dynamics manifest through majority and minority groups, market forces, and political interests. Beneficence, respect for persons, social utility, and justice (distributive and procedural), as well as non-maleficence (first of all, do no harm) are moral norms that emerge frequently, if tacitly, in the pages that follow, whether as rationales *for* resistance, as warrants for interventions *in spite of* resistance, or as considerations when practitioners and local communities dialogue regarding *which* public health interventions are most suitable.

In situations where a proposed public health intervention involves a conflict between two or more competing ethical norms, overriding one or more of these moral norms requires ethical justification (see Childress, 2015). Such ethical justification involves giving an account for the intervention as proposed in light of the potential modifications that might be made to the proposed or alternative interventions. In order to justify overriding ethical norms where two or more norms conflict, one must consider several aspects of the proposed intervention, including its likelihood of success, whether it is the least infringement necessary, the proportionality of benefits and burdens, and the impartiality in how these benefits and burdens are distributed. Consider, for example, the following questions: Likelihood of success: Is there a reasonable prospect of success such that the intervention under consideration warrants overriding the liberty, privacy, confidentiality, or other expressed wishes of the affected parties? Least infringement: Is there an alternative intervention that involves less coercive means and that is likely to produce comparable public health outcomes? Proportionality: Do the benefits of an intervention outweigh its negative effects to a sufficient degree so as to justify overriding the other moral norms involved? Impartiality: Does the proposed intervention avoid discriminating biases, and does it attend to the concerns of vulnerable, stigmatized, and marginalized groups? Holding public health interventions accountable to these considerations serves to lessen, and sometimes to remove, ethically objectionable or undesirable burdens that are often features of public health interventions. Of course, ethical justification requires not only that the above considerations and questions be addressed but also, and perhaps most importantly, fairness in terms of who gets to participate in raising objections and weighing the various moral considerations.

Whereas distributive justice attends to proportionality and impartiality in how the benefits and burdens of public health interventions are distributed across a population, procedural justice attends to issues of transparency, inclusion, and revisability. In short, a just process includes a publicly articulated, ongoing exchange of reasons among all interested and impacted parties for the interventions under consideration. Transparency in such a process includes disclosure of the potentially conflicting interests as well as continual public access to public health priorities, decision-making policies and procedures, and community health surveillance data and trends. Inclusion refers to the participation of the affected community members and institutions and their concerns in the policy-making process. It requires not only an openness to those who voice concerns, but an active seeking out of those voices all too often silenced or disenfranchised by structural biases built into cultural patterns of exclusion. Revisability ensures the continued involvement of the affected parties as the public health situation evolves over time. As situations change, public health interventions may prove more or less successful, new information and medical treatments become available, and the (re)emergence of new and old diseases can greatly effect the priorities of different constituencies within a population. As a result, prior determinations regarding public health priorities and interventions remain in principle revisable through an ongoing conversation among the relevant stakeholders that is both transparent and inclusive. Because the justifiability of interventions is not static but ever changing as individuals' and groups' needs and interests evolve, procedural justice demands transparency, inclusion, and revisability in determining priorities, implementation of procedures, and ongoing reassessment of interventions.

Critical medical anthropology scholarship has long presented itself as much more than a descriptive discipline, and in this volume, our contributors continue that tradition as we advocate for certain approaches to public health interventions as more ethically justifiable than others. To the degree that we make normative judgments and engage in normative ethics, our aim is to exercise our critical gaze upon these normative commitments that are operative in our second-order reflection upon public health.

The case studies in this volume reflect the relative successes and failures of public health interventions to attend to the manifold of ethical considerations that are deemed significant by the various stakeholders involved. Each chapter offers a distinct vantage from which to observe how individuals and communities have attempted to understand, negotiate, and justify their own and others' responses to real and perceived interests and moral obligations. In some cases, the ethical considerations rise to the surface and are made explicit; for example, in Gottlieb's discussion of Gardasil vaccination policies and Peterson and colleagues' portrayal of pharmaceutical trials in Nigeria and Malawi. In others, readers will discern unarticulated, implicit ethical concerns operative in defiance to public health interventions in ways that, we hope, bring additional, significant aspects of the cases into relief.

Resisting public health strategies

Throughout history, communities have protested against the intrusion of biomedically based public health efforts. These acts, whether limited to casual conversation, or organized as individual intentions or social movements, continue to take place across the world. Their rationales differ, as do their outcomes. A superficial examination of these disruptions might indicate an unwillingness to accept new knowledge, new strategies, or new technologies. The new might appear in conflict with the established. A conflict of culture is often cited as the cause of disruptions, and a failing of public health practitioners to recognize, understand, and alter the approach to accommodate to new cultural contexts. In some cases, this may indeed be the cause of conflict. However, as this collection will reveal, deeper issues are often being negotiated through these acts of defiance.

For example, in colonial Africa, public health teams seeking to eradicate sleeping sickness by extracting lymph fluid from the neck of suspected patients were consciously avoided. In the Belgian Congo, people would flee into the bush to escape the mobile public health disease eradication teams, or persuade traditional physicians to remove their lymph nodes so that they would not be subjected to the dreaded needles (Lyons, 1988, 1992). Europeans' viewed the introduction of scientific enquiry and biomedicine as a central feature of their 'gift' of civilization to Africans. However, this came with a harsh, repressive political system, a ruthlessly exploitative economic system, and the introduction of new diseases and exacerbation and spread of existing diseases (Lyons, 1992). Resistance on the part of indigenous populations to comply with the practices of colonial medicine suggests not just a conflict of healing beliefs and practices or a fear of unknown biomedical practices, but opposition to the authority of colonial rulers. Luise White (2000) has shown how vampire rumors in East Africa were a powerful local commentary on colonialism, offering a vivid imagery of bloodsucking Europeans.

Vaccines have commonly aroused public concerns. Vaccinations for various diseases became compulsory for infants up to 3 months old in the U.K. in 1853 (Drake et al., 2001). The smallpox vaccine received considerable resistance from parents as the process involved scoring the flesh on a child's forearm and inserting lymph from the blister formed at the vaccination site of an individual who had been vaccinated about a week earlier. Objections to vaccinations related to religious ideology, distrust of medicine, suspicions over efficacy, and violations of personal liberties (Durbach, 2000). In the U.K., the Anti-Vaccination League and the Anti-Compulsory Vaccination League formed in response to mandatory laws (Wolfe & Sharpe, 2002). By 1898, public demonstrations and general opposition resulted in a revised Vaccination Act that removed penalties for parents who did not want to submit their child(ren) to vaccination, adding a "conscientious objector" clause and an exemption certificate (Wolfe & Sharpe, 2002).

Smallpox outbreaks in the U.S. similarly spurred mandatory vaccine efforts and corresponding public resistance. The Anti-Vaccination Society of America and the New England Anti-Compulsory Vaccination League, along with other anti-vaccine groups, were established in the late 1800s, prompted by activist movements in the U.K. A smallpox outbreak in Cambridge, Massachusetts, in 1902 resulted in mandatory vaccination. In a precedent setting public health law case, Cambridge city resident Henning Jacobson refused vaccination on grounds that the law violated his right to care for his own body. After many years of legal battles, in 1905 the U.S. Supreme Court found in favor of the state, ruling that in public health emergencies, the state could establish mandatory rulings to protect the public from communicable disease (Albert, Ostheimer, & Breman, 2001; Gostin, 2005).

Public resistance to vaccines continues to be a major public health concern today. In the U.S., resistance to childhood vaccinations, which has reduced vaccination coverage levels needed to achieve herd or social immunity, contributed to the 2014 'Disneyland' measles outbreak that consequently spread nationally. Similar outbreaks occurred in Canada, countries in Europe, Asia, and Oceana. According to the WHO, 110 measles deaths were reported in the Philippines in 2014, and most of the over 21,000 confirmed cases of measles were in unvaccinated people. The newly developed Human Papilloma Vaccine (HPV) has seen resistance sparked in different ways and among different populations in the U.S. and Japan (see Gottlieb's chapter in this volume and Parpia, 2015). These parental concerns are not necessarily consistent with the concerns of the public in places were infectious diseases remain a major killer of children. International donor and aid agencies are often determining how best to address these concerns (Closser et al., 2014; Leach & Fairhead, 2007).

Explorations of vaccine resistance in developing nations reveal a complex interplay of history and politics, religion, the context of the broader health system, and the delivery of immunizations themselves (Closser et al., 2014; Feldman-Savelsberg, Ndonko, & Schmidt-Ehry, 2000; Ghinai, Willott, Dadari, & Larson, 2013; Nichter, 1995; Streefland, 2001). Several scholars have noted that historical efforts by colonial governments to vaccinate indigenous populations (Anderson, 2006; Neill, 2012) continue to influence contemporary vaccination campaigns (Arnold, 1993; Feldman-Savelsberg et al., 2000; Hardon, 2004). Memories also influence more recent vaccination efforts, as seen in Nigeria, where memories of the 1996 Pfizer's Trovan meningitis drug treatment trials, during which 11 children died, colored conversations about the polio vaccine (Ghinai et al., 2013; Larson, Cooper, Eskola, Katz, & Ratzan, 2011; Yahya, 2007).

Local and global politics, including distrust of Western powers perceived to be behind vaccination programs (Feldman-Savelsberg et al., 2000; Nichter, 1995) also stimulate vaccine refusal. Polio vaccine refusals in Nigeria have been attributed to political tensions within the country, to patron-clientism fueled by the relatively deep pockets of polio prevention efforts, and a distrust of U.S. intervention (Ghinai et al., 2013; Larson et al., 2011; Leach & Fairhead, 2007; Yahya, 2007). Some research suggests that groups that are physically or socially marginalized are more likely to refuse vaccines (Das, Das, & Coutinho, 2000). Alternatively, local acceptance appears influenced by the delivery of the immunization or the quality of the immunization program overall (Coutinho & Banerjea, 2000; Das et al., 2000; Feldman-Savelsberg et al., 2000; Greenough, 1995; Hardon, 2004; Larson et al., 2011; Nichter, 1995; Streefland, 2001; Streefland, Chowdhury, & Ramos-Jimenez, 1999; Yahya, 2007). While it may seem logical that efficient, high-quality vaccination programs with trustworthy and respected staff improves public acceptance of vaccination efforts, research indicates that community members can be suspicious of well-organized, well-funded campaigns, particularly when other local health services remain disorganized and of poor quality (Closser et al., 2014; Closser et al., 2015).

While resistance to vaccines has a long history and is both well organized and well publicized, other resistance efforts have been less documented, and thus, while no less important, less considered. For example, the introduction of fluoride to community water supplies, although heralded by the U.S. Centers for Disease Control and Prevention as one of the "Ten Great Public Health Achievements" of the past century (CDC, 1999), has been contested by members of the public. A large anti-fluoridation subculture has developed arguing against the public health intervention to prevent dental caries citing economic, medical, environmental, and ethical concerns (Freeze & Lehr, 2009). Detractors have noted the possibility of undesirable and highly damaging side effects, including cancer, birth defects, osteoarthritis, osteoporosis, bone fracture, kidney disease, premature aging, allergies, Alzheimer's disease, and heart disease (Corbin, 1989; Pollick, 2004). They also cite a lack of public health necessity, given alternatives that are both sufficient and less intrusive, such as fluoride treatments and toothpaste (Balog, 1997). Yet these alternatives are not universally available, as discussed by Sarah Horton and Judith Barker in this volume. Without fluoridation and the public will to provide funding for alternatives, vulnerable populations benefiting the most from this strategy would suffer. The case of anti-fluoridation efforts highlights the need for public health policy to involve more than just utilitarian assessments of financial and public health risks and benefits. Procedural justice demands that public health strategies involve continued and intentional communication that ensures the public's involvement in decisions.

These selected accounts of disruption as mentioned here, from early vaccine campaigns to recent efforts to contain a potential global Ebola outbreak, reveal the struggles incumbent in public health efforts. The intent in pointing out resistance is not to suggest that public health efforts are all inappropriately imposed by outsiders and ethically concerning. Rather, accounts of disruption highlight the difficulties inherent in public health work, as the struggles between individual rights and common good are constantly negotiated, as history informs the present, as new ideas, approaches, and technologies are understood in different ways, and as global and local politics and economics generate divisions that are contested through the everyday and often overlooked efforts.

Organization of the book

This collection thinks through cases of resistance to contemporary global public health strategies, with a particular focus on those strategies dependent on technologies (i.e., vaccines, surgeries, pharmaceuticals, dentistry, and toilets). The theoretical frame of critical medical anthropology is used as a way to explore the historical, political, and economic foundations of expertise, subjugation, resistance, and reconfiguration. The following questions guide each case:

- What catalyzes movements of opposition toward health interventions?
- What characterizes resistance and, by contrast, effective integration and acceptance of useful interventions?
- Can examining resistance help global health practitioners anticipate potential problems as they develop and implement new interventions and alternative strategies?
- What does resistance indicate about the contemporary state of global health governance?
- What can the critical medical anthropology perspective contribute to reimaging global health in the context of health intervention resistance?

This collection aims to highlight important critiques of current global health practice, by employing and advancing the theoretical perspective of critical medical anthropology. The collection addresses global inequities and the role of global public health institutions in perpetuating these inequities. Specifically, authors of this collection consider the two focal points of global health programs: the focus on individuals as rational decision makers, whose characteristics or capacities predict health outcomes; and the consideration of structural vulnerabilities, such as poverty, as a predictor of behavior and health outcomes for entire populations (Singer, 2015). These approaches have resulted in technocratic vertical programming, universalization, concerns over cost-effectiveness, rather than the identification of effective and sustainable solutions, the imposition of ideas founded in 'science' and developed by outside experts, and the development of governing strategies that limit both the involvement of locals and the opportunity for dialogue. The relationship between individual agency and structural factors in health is not considered. As such, resistance, whether as organized collectives, or as personal decisions not to engage, serves as a form of advocacy calling for changes in global health structures, local health-care delivery, and expanded access to social programs, infrastructure, and medical technologies that will offer more significant improvements in the overall health of individuals and populations.

In pulling together these case studies on resistance to public health efforts, the aim is not to simply offer a critique and restate what is already well accepted – that the world is full of inequity and sometimes the best-intended efforts to address this only make it worse. Rather, we take up the challenge put forth by James Ferguson (2011), who offered insights on the use of Foucauldian models of analyses to critique power (in our case, institutions of public health). Ferguson suggests that too often "power has been 'critiqued,' an oppressive system has been exposed. . .[illuminating revelations are made that] the current world system. . .rests on inequality and exploitation. . . . But such lines of argument typically have very little to propose by way of an alternative 'art of government'" (2011, p. 62). This volume draws together a collection of cases (of experiments) that, while highlighting global inequity and revealing global public health institutions as a form of governing, think through resistance and denunciations of power as a way of proposing alternative forms of governing. The moments of resistance examined call for an alternative approach to global public health, a reimagining of sorts, that extends beyond greater distribution of medical technologies to one that articulates and builds on the perspectives of a political economy of health.

The chapters that follow are all individual cases of disruption to public health policy or programming. The chapters are purposefully geographically and topically diverse, highlighting the key concerns of global public health today, which relate to specific diseases, technologies, and policy development strategies. Each case contributes to the creation of a single argument – the need for a new approach to global public health. Taken together, they provide a kaleidoscopic view of the terrain of opportunities. In Chapter 2, Mohan Dutta and Ambar Basu draw on their culture-centered fieldwork in West Bengal, India, and Singapore to offer a perspective on public health communication as representative of broader global structures, explore the theoretical framework of 'culture-centered' approaches, and indicate the varied forms of resistance (as memory, as talk, as everyday acts, as collective participation) that take shape. In Chapter 3, Samantha Gottlieb returns us to discussions of vaccine refusal, but with a new twist in her examination of U.S. state considerations to mandate Gardasil, the first vaccine for human papillomavirus (HPV), as part of school entry requirements. In Chapter 4, Alex Nading takes us to Nicaragua where mosquito control efforts against dengue fever are complicated by the efforts of vulnerable populations to secure an economic livelihood. In Chapter 5, Nicola Bulled and Edward C. Green explore the acceptance of (or lack thereof) the new HIV prevention technology – voluntary medical male circumcision – in Swaziland and Lesotho. In Chapter 6, Kristin Peterson, Morenike Oluwatoyin Folayan, Edward Chigwedere, and Evaristo Nthete examine the ethics of clinical trials related to another new HIV prevention technology – pre-exposure prophylaxis (PrEP) – in Malawi and Nigeria. In Chapter 7, Sarah Horton and Judith Barker relay the concerns of Latino immigrant children as they struggle with both the stigma related to poor dental health and limited access to dental health care in the U.S. state of California. In Chapter 8, Christopher Colvin and Steven Robins offer a discussion of organized resistance to state public health programming and policy as they compare and contrast three social movement organizations in South Africa.

Together these cases reveal that public health programing and biomedical technologies are most often not the object of resistance. In addition, fear, uncertainty, and cultural differences in illness causality (and consequently prevention and treatment) are not the prime motivations of resistance. As evident in these cases, disruptions to the state/global public health agenda reveal that technologies and innovations are often desired. Resistance calls attention to the inequitable distribution of these technologies, challenges established notions of self-responsibilized health and liberal individualist conceptions of 'proper citizenship,' and questions citizen-state relationships and the power differences that the technocratic approach perpetuates between those who devise solutions (experts) and those who receive them. The authors present interpretations of contemporary public health efforts that emphasize the agency of ordinary people, and their ability to disrupt the everyday operations of power and authority. The results of these disruptions are however, unpredictable.

Collectively, this volume fleshes out the bare framework of an argument for a new global health structure. We challenge readers to consider how these examinations of resistance to contemporary public health efforts might offer a guide to imagine a different approach to public health policy and programming. Perhaps we might adopt what Hans Joas (2013) has termed an "affirmative genealogy" approach, in considering every individual as sacred in the pursuit of population level goals. Or, we might look to the economist William Easterly (2013), who has proposed a celebration of "spontaneous solutions" rather than a reliance on the illusion of "conscious design" as a way to accept that while an approach works in one area it should not be considered appropriate for another. Similarly, we should consider the concept of "asset based public health," a look to celebrating and building upon existing elements as a step toward a new possibility in global public health efforts.

References

Albert, M., Ostheimer, K., & Breman, J. (2001). The last smallpox epidemic in Boston and the vaccination controversy. *New England Journal of Medicine, 344*(5), 375–379.

Ammann, T. (2014). Ebola in Liberia: A threat to human security and peace. *Fieldsights – Hot Spots, Cultural Anthropology Online.*

Anderson, W. (2006). *Colonial Pathologies: American Tropical Medicine, Race, and Hygiene in the Philippines.* Durham, NC: Duke University Press.

Arnold, D. (1993). *Colonizing the Body: State Medicine and Epidemic Disease in Nineteenth-Century India.* Berkeley: University of California Press.

Ashton, J., & Ubido, J. (1991). The healthy city and the ecological idea. *Journal of the Society for the Social History of Medicine, 4*(1), 173–181. doi:10.1093/shm/4.1.173

Balog, D.A. (1997). Fluoridation of public water systems: Valid exercise of state police power or constitutional violation? *Pace Environmental Law Review, 14*(2), Paper 314.

Barry, G., & Carruthers, L. A. (2005). *A History of Britain's Hospitals.* East Sussex: The Book Guild Ltd.

Batty, F. (2014). Reinventing "others" in a time of Ebola. Hot Spots, *Cultural Anthropology*, October 7, 2014. https://culanth.org/fieldsights/589-reinventing-others-in-a-time-of-ebola.

Bellah, R. N. (2011). *Religion in Human Evolution: From the Paleolithic to the Axial Age.* Cambridge, MA: Harvard University Press.

Birn, A., & Solórzano, A. (1999). Public health policy paradoxes: Science and politics in the Rockefeller Foundation's hookworm campaign in Mexico in the 1920s. *Social Science & Medicine, 49*(9), 1197. doi:10.1016/S0277-9536(99)00160-4

Brown, J. (2015). *South Africa's Insurgent Citizens: On Dissent and the Possibility of Politics.* Auckland Park, South Africa: Jacana Media.

Carbone, S. (1962). Superintendents and Sopraprovveditori of Health of the Republic of Venice. Inventory Rome: Correspondence with diplomatic and consular representatives abroad and with Venetian offices of foreign correspondents Health. Notebooks of the Review of the State Archives, 21.

CDC. (1999). Ten great public health achievements – United States, 1900–1999. *Morbidity and Mortality Weekly Report, 48*(12), 241–243.

Chaplin, J. (2001). *Subject Matter: Technology, the Body, and Science on the Anglo-American Frontier, 1500–1676.* Cambridge: Harvard University Press.

Childress, J. F. (2015). Moral considerations: Bases and limits for public health interventions. In R. G. Bernheim, J. F. Childress, R. J. Bonnie, & A. L. Melnick (Eds.), *Essentials of Public Health Ethics*. Burlington, MA: Jones & Bartlett.

Childress, J. F., & Bernheim, R. G. (2008). Public health ethics: Public justification and public trust. *Bundesgesundheitsblatt, Gesundheitsforschung, Gesundheitsschutz, 51*(2), 158–163.

Closser, S., Cox, K., Parris, T., Landis, R., Justice, J., Gopinath, R., . . . Nuttall, E. (2014). The impact of polio eradication on routine immunization and primary health care: A mixed-methods study. *Journal of Infectious Disease, 210 Suppl 1*, S504-513. doi:10.1093/infdis/jit232

Closser, S., Rosenthal, A., Maes, K., Justic, J., Cox, K., Omidian, P., . . . Koon, A. (2015). The global context of vaccine refusal: Insights from a systematic comparative ethnography of the global polio eradication initiative. *Medical Anthropology Quarterly*. [epub ahead of print] doi:10.1111/maq.12229

Corbin, S. B. (1989). Fluoridation then and now. *American Journal of Public Health, 79*(5), 561–563.

Coutinho, L., & Banerjea, N. (2000). Social production of blame: Case study of OPV-related deaths in West Bengal. *Economic and Political Weekly, 35*(8/9), 709–717.

da Mosto, A. (n.d.). The State Archives of Venice. Contents, historical, descriptive and analytics. Retrieved from http://www.archiviodistatovenezia.it/web/

Das, V., Das, R. K., & Coutinho, L. (2000). Disease control and immunisation: A sociological enquiry. *Economic and Political Weekly, 35*(8/9), 625–632.

Douglas, M. (2002 [1966]). *Purity and Danger: An Analysis of Concepts of Pollution and Taboo.* London: Routledge.

Drake, M., Razzell, M., Rider, J., Hack, J., Birch, P., Walsh, J., . . . Fellows, C. (2001). Decline of Infant Mortality in England and Wales, 1871–1948: A Medical Conundrum. doi:10.5255/UKDA-SN-4127-1

Durbach, N. (2000). 'They might as well brand us': Working-class resistance to compulsory vaccination in Victorian England. *The Society for the Social History of Medicine, 13*, 45–62.

Easterly, W. (2013). *The Tyranny of Experts: Economists, Dictators, and the Forgotten Rights of the Poor*. New York: Basic Books.

Fa-hsien, & Legge, J. (1886). *A Record of Buddhistic Kingdoms being an Account by the Chinese Monk of his Travels in India and Ceylon (A.D. 399–414) in Search of the Buddhist Books of Discipline*. Oxford, UK: Clarendon Press.

Fassin, D. (2007). *When Bodies Remember: Experiences and Politics of AIDS in South Africa.* Berkeley, CA: University of California Press.

Feldman-Savelsberg, P., Ndonko, F. T., & Schmidt-Ehry, B. (2000). Sterilizing vaccines or the politics of the womb: Retrospective study of a rumor in Cameroon. *Medical Anthropology Quarterly, 14*(2), 159–179.

Ferguson, J. (2011). Toward a left art of government: From 'Foucauldian critique' to Foucauldian politics. *History of the Human Sciences, 24*(4), 61–68. doi:10.1177/0952695111413849

Fink, S. (2014). Cuts at WHO Hurt Response to Ebola Crisis. *New York Times*. Retrieved from http://www.nytimes.com/2014/09/04/world/africa/cuts-at-who-hurt-response-to-ebola-crisis.html

Foucault, M. (2010). *The Birth of Biopolitics: Lectures at the College de France, 1978–1979*. New York: Picador.

Freeze, R. A., & Lehr, J. H. (2009). *The Fluoride Wars: How a Modest Health Measure Became America's Longest-Running Political Melodrama*. Hoboken, NJ: John Wiley & Sons.

Garrett, L. (2015). Ebola's lessons: How the WHO mishandled the crisis. *Foreign Affairs, September/October*. https://www.foreignaffairs.com/articles/west-africa/2015-08-18/ebolas-lessons?campaign=Garrett.

Ghinai, I., Willott, C., Dadari, I., & Larson, H. (2013). Listening to the rumours: What the northern Nigeria polio vaccine boycott can tell us ten years on. *Global Public Health, 8*(10), 1138–1150. doi:10.1080/17441692.2013.859720

Gostin, L. (2005). Jacobson vs. Massachusetts at 100 years: Police powers and civil liberties in tension. *American Journal of Public Health, 95*, 576–581.

Greene, J., Basilico, M. T., Kim, H., & Farmer, P. (2013). Colonial medicine and its legacies. In P. Farmer, J. Y. Kim, A. Kleinman, & M. Basilico (Eds.), *Reimagining Global Health: An Introduction* (pp. 33–73). Berkeley: University of California Press.

Greenough, P. (1995). Intimidation, coercion and resistance in the final stages of the South Asian Smallpox Eradication Campaign, 1973–1975. *Social Science & Medicine, 41*(5), 633–645.

Hardon, A. (2004). *Immunization: Global Programs, Local Acceptance and Resistance. In Encyclopedia of Medical Anthropology: Health and Illness in the World's Cultures*. New York: Springer.

Horton, S. B., & Barker, J. C. (2009). "Stains" on their self-discipline: Public health, hygiene, and the disciplining of undocumented immigrant parents in the nation's internal borderlands. *American Ethnologist, 36*(4), 784–798. doi:10.1111/j.1548-1425.2009.01210.x

Joas, H. (2013). *The Sacredness of the Person: A New Genealogy of Human Rights*. Georgetown: Georgetown University Press.

Jones, D. (2004). *Rationalizing Epidemics*. Cambridge: Harvard University Press.

Larson, H., Cooper, L., Eskola, J., Katz, S., & Ratzan, S. (2011). Addressing the vaccine confidence gap. *Lancet, 378*(9790), 526–535. doi:10.1016/S0140-6736(11)60678-8

Leach, M., & Fairhead, J. (2007). *Vaccine Anxieties: Global Science, Child Health, and Society*. Oxon, UK: Earthscan

Leibniz, G. (1952). *Theodicy: Essays on the Goodness of God, the Freedom of Man and the Origin of Evil*. (E. Huggard, Trans.). A. Farrer (Ed.). New Haven: Yale University Press.

Lyons, M. (1988). Sleeping sickness, colonial medicine and imperialism: Some connections in the Belgian Congo. In R. Macleod & L. Milton (Eds.), *Disease, Medicine and Empire* (pp. 242–256). London, UK: Routledge.

Lyons, M. (1992). *The Colonial Disease: A Social History of Sleeping Sickness in Northern Zaire, 1900–1940*. Cambridge: Cambridge University Press.

Mooney, G. (2015). *Intrusive Interventions: Public Health, Domestic Space, and Infectious Disease Surveillance in England, 1840–1914*. Rochester, NY: University of Rochester Press.

Moran, M., & Hoffman, D. (2014). Introduction: Ebola in perspective. Hot Spots, *Cultural Anthropology,* October 7, 2014. https://culanth.org/fieldsights/586-introduction-ebola-in-perspective.

Neill, D. J. (2012). *Networks in Tropical Medicine: Internationalism, Colonialism, and the Rise of a Medical Specialty 1890–1930*. Stanford: Stanford University Press.

Nichter, M. (1995). Vaccinations in the Third World: A consideration of community demand. *Social Science & Medicine, 41*(5), 617–632.

Nossiter, A. (2014). Fear of Ebola Breeds a Terror of Physicians. *New York Times*. Retrieved from http://www.nytimes.com/2014/07/28/world/africa/ebola-epidemic-west-africa-guinea.html

Parpia, R. (2015). Japan, U.S. Poles Apart on Harmful HPV Vaccine. *The Vaccine Reaction*. Retrieved from http://www.thevaccinereaction.org/2015/06/japan-u-s-poles-apart-on-harmful-hpv-vaccine/

Paul, B. D. (Ed.) (1955). *Health, Culture and Community: Case Studies of Public Reactions to Health Programs*. New York, NY: Russel Sage Foundations.

Pepin, J. (2011). *The Origins of AIDS*. Cambridge, UK: Cambridge University Press.

Pollick, H. F. (2004). Water fluoridation and the environment: Current perspective in the United States. *International Journal of Occupational Environmental Health, 10*, 343–350.

Rhodes, P. (2015). Public health. *Encyclopaedia Britannica*. Chicago.

Risse, G. B. (1999). *Mending Bodies, Saving Souls: A History of Hospitals*. New York: Oxford University Press.

Schroven, A. (2014). Ebola in Guinea: Revealing the state of the state. Hot Spots, *Cultural Anthropology*, October 7, 2014. https://culanth.org/fieldsights/587-ebola-in-guinea-revealing-the-state-of-the-state.

Singer, M. (2015). *Anthropology of Infectious Disease*. Walnut Creek: Left Coast Press.

Streefland, P. (2001). Public doubts about vaccination safety and resistance against vaccination. *Health Policy, 55*(3), 159–172.

Streefland, P., Chowdhury, A., & Ramos-Jimenez, P. (1999). Quality of vaccination services and social demand for vaccinations in Africa and Asia. *Bulletin of the World Health Organization*, 77(9), 722–730.

Swanson, M. W. (1977). The sanitation syndrome: Bubonic plague and urban native policy in the Cape Colony, 1900–1909. *Journal of African History, 18*(3), 387–410.

Voltaire. (2005). The Lisbon earthquake. In *Candide, or Optimism* (T. Smollett, Trans.). London: Penguin Books.

White, L. (2000). *Speaking with Vampires: Rumor and History in Colonial Africa*. Berkeley, CA: University of California Press.

Wilken, R. L. (2012). The sick, the aged, and the poor: The birth of hospitals. In *The First Thousand Years: A Global History of Christianity* (pp. 154–162). New Haven: Yale University Press.

Wolfe, R., & Sharpe, L. (2002). Anti-vaccinationists past and present. *British Medical Journal, 325*, 430–432.

Worboys, M. (1976). The emergence of tropical medicine. In G. Lemaine, R. Macleod, M. Mulkay, & P. Weingart (Eds.), *Perspective on the Emergency of Scientific Disciplines* (pp. 82–85). London: Routledge.

Yahya, M. (2007). Polio Vaccines – "no Thank You!" Barriers to Polio Eradication in Northern Nigeria. *African Affairs, 106*(423), 185–204.

2

SUBALTERN RESISTANCE NARRATIVES AND THE CULTURE-CENTERED APPROACH

Inverting Public Health Discourse

Mohan J. Dutta and Ambar Basu

In 1948, the World Health Organization defined health as a "state of complete physical, mental and social well-being and not merely the absence of disease or infirmity" (WHO, 1948). However, researchers note that over the years, conceptualizations of health and illness in marginalized Third World spaces continue to operate under the ambit of the Western biomedical paradigm of prevention and individual psychology-driven behavior change (C. Airhihenbuwa & Obregon, 2000; C. O. Airhihenbuwa, 1995; Dutta-Bergman, 2005; Dutta, 2008; Lupton, 1994). This model erases health narratives that materialize in subaltern spaces around the globe. These erased narratives are often noteworthy in the ways they are framed and acted out as texts that resist the dominant public health discourse. In this chapter, we present these narratives of resistance. We draw from several culture-centered fieldwork sites to make our argument. In the first half of the chapter, we position the culture-centered approach in the light of the dominant public health communication paradigm. In the second half, subaltern stories of resistance to this dominant paradigm are presented.

Public health communication as representation of the broader structures

Lupton (1994) writes that the dominant/Western paradigm or the mainstream biomedical paradigm of public health is tied to notions of development and globalization. It endorses claims to power over the human body, which is construed as a domain of knowledge, as a carrier of health and disease, to be controlled, corrected, and improved on by organized centers of power in society (Foucault, 1984; Lupton, 2003; Nandy, 1988). Nandy notes: "Development is no more development unless it takes the benefits of modern medicine to the traditional, underdeveloped parts of society, unless diseases and pestilences are removed, by modern knowledge, from the lives of the citizens" (1988, p. 146). Airhihenbuwa notes that the logic of globalization as the "new language of universal truth" (1995, p. xi) continues to feed on the need to transform and civilize the wretched of the earth (Fanon, 1968), continuing to focus on individual behavior change and thus obliterating the need to transform structures that create conditions of marginality (Dutta, 2008). This exacerbates inequities between the haves and the have-nots in terms of access to resources and communicative platforms that promote health and well-being. Culture, context, and social structures are taken out of the construction of the human body. The body becomes a subject of pathological systematic imbalances that can be corrected using modern techniques and medicinal procedures.

Deborah Lupton (2003) states that the dominant public health discourse constructs health at the level of individual responsibility, whereby every person is responsible for his/her health, disease states, and well-being. A diseased individual is labeled as deviant and is liable to be sanctioned and corrected by those who are given power by the medical system. In this process, the cultural production of health and the function of modern medicine become methods of social control and surveillance (Foucault, 1984). The onus of being responsible for one's health resides on the individual, opening up communicative spaces that engender labeling of the "irresponsible" as deviant and justifying the need to correct and civilize him or her through interventions designed in the "rational," more "civilized" West (Lupton, 2003).

Needless to say, such interventions are rooted in the agenda of the biomedical model of health and behavior change. This model emphasizes the transmission of beliefs, information, and knowledge via one-way health messages from the core sectors of the globe to spaces in the periphery, based on the assumption of the expert position of the sender of the message. The notion driving this dominant approach to global public health promotion is that the expert knows what is best for the passive receivers. Summarizing the essence of such mainstream top-down health communication efforts, Lupton states that members of target populations in marginalized spaces are often regarded as "apathetic and ignorant, needful of persuasion to change their behavior, resistant to change, obstinate, recalcitrant, lacking self-efficacy, and chronically uninformed" (1994, p. 56). Dutta-Bergman (2005) argues that these interventions are political exercises dictated by those in power that "select and frame social conditions and groups as problematic, legitimizing particular approaches to their resolution and not others" (Wilkins & Mody, 2001, p. 393). The primary objective of such public health initiatives, he adds, is persuasion, and the epistemological premise of such efforts is based on a "desire for control and domination" (Foss & Griffin, 1995, p. 3). This individual-centered orientation, Airhihenbuwa (2007) argues, in the realm of HIV/AIDS, engenders the "formation of a generation of managers of human behavior and technocrats and administrators of the epidemic who have provided us with elegant but acultural and acontextual recipes" (p. 150) for judging what is framed as risky or deviant behaviors.

This top-down model normalizes the health behavior prescribed by a campaign such that if it fails, the target community is painted as deficient, lacking in knowledge, skill, and/or motivation to put expert advice into practice; the interventionists absolve themselves of any accountability for the failure of the program. Absent in the articulation of such public health discourses are factors such as socioeconomic status, access to resources, cultural and community norms, and issues related to race, class, and gender. By not accounting for these factors, the dominant knowledge creation apparatus backgrounds the need to alter and challenge structures that marginalize (Dutta, 2008). Also absent are the participatory practices of members of communities who are at the heart of such campaign efforts (Dutta, 2008). Subalternity is thus produced at sites of public health communication efforts, constituting the erasures of subaltern voices through expert-led top-down public health efforts.

The term "subalternity," John Beverly (2004) notes, refers to a condition of subordination brought about by colonization (in its past and contemporary formations) or other forms of economic, social, cultural, racial, and/or linguistic dominance. The Subaltern Studies project began with the work of Ranajit Guha and the South Asian Subaltern Studies collective in the 1980s in response to what Guha describes as "disillusionment of hope" at the failure of the Indian nation state to fulfill its "promise of nationhood even two decades after Britain's retreat" (1997, p. xii). Subaltern Studies, Beverly points out, is about power, about "who has it and who doesn't, who is gaining it and who is losing it" (Beverly, 2004, p. 1). It is a project of positioning the subaltern with respect to her/his condition of colonialilty, a condition that peripheralizes her/him to the margins of modern civil society and its processes of knowledge creation and writing history.

Extended to the realm of public health initiatives, Subaltern Studies creates entry points for listening to the histories and the voices of subalterns as they script their localized vocabularies on health, illness, and suffering. Existing literature that connects the Subaltern Studies project to health programs documents, for example, how sex workers organize to fight institutional and structural violence in order to retrieve access to monetary capacities that augment their ability to stay healthy and safe from HIV/AIDS (Basu, 2011; Basu & Dutta, 2008, 2011).

The culture-centered approach is set up in response to and as a paradigmatic shift from this dominant ideology that informs most public health efforts (Dutta, 2008). It underlines the understanding that communicating about and practicing healthy behaviors is essentially a process of negotiation of shared meanings situated in interdependent notions of culture, identities, social norms, and structures.

Culture-centered approach: Invitation to listen

Privileging the narratives that emerge through conversations with members of marginalized communities, the culture-centered approach highlights the interaction between culture, structure, and agency in how health is theorized at the margins (Dutta, 2008). While structures constrain and limit the possibilities of health among underserved people, agency is enacted in its interaction with the structures and embodies communicative actions and processes that challenge, navigate, and attempt to change these structures. This line of thinking foregrounds the importance of understanding articulations of health by engaging local cultural enunciations and thus presents opportunities for social change by documenting narratives of resistance at the margins to expert-led public health initiatives and dominant articulations of social reality and cultural and behavioral norms.

Culture, structure, and agency

Culture can be defined as the communicative process of production and reconfiguration of webs of shared meanings, beliefs, practices, and rituals (Geertz, 1973; Helman, 1986). It comprises the social, economic, and political webs encompassing values that influence attitudes, perceptions, and communication behaviors in a society (C. O. Airhihenbuwa, 1995). Culture can be construed as the living framework of individuals and their collectives – a learned/learning experience, a process of evolving, living, learning, adapting, orienting, thinking, communicating, and producing knowledge within which individuals and social groups operate (Ford & Yep, 2003). Culture in this sense is transitive, shifting its meanings based on the nature of the situation and the evolving processes of sense-making that cultural participants engage in. The culture-centered approach stresses on the need to theorize and practice public health practices that are consistent with people's cultural frameworks. The goal in such an approach is not to extract cultural characteristics of a targeted population and predict how such characteristics vary with patterns of health communication. Rather, the goal is to listen to how communities living at the margins of society make meanings on health and illness and accommodate those narratives and values into public health efforts targeted at the community.

Structure refers to forms of social organizing that provide or limit access to resources (Dutta, 2008). These resources script human behavior that guide culture and conduct. Structures define and limit the possibilities that are available to cultural participants as they enact agency to engage in practices that influence their health and well-being. Structures that influence health include those at the micro-level, like community medical services, community modes of transportation, channels of communication, and health-enhancing resources such as food, clean spaces, and spaces for exercising; meso-level resources such as points of policy implementation, avenues of civil society organizations, and media platforms; and macro-level resources such as national and international political actors and points of policy formulation and national and global health organizations (Basu & Dutta, 2008; Dutta, 2008). Structures at these multiple levels work in tandem to influence each other and the health outcomes of participants who create and reify such structures as well as engage with them to create discursive webs that frame their lives. The emphasis in the culture-centered approach is to gain an understanding of these structures that limit the possibilities of health for members of a community.

For the homeless, for instance, structural barriers that impede access to use of health-care facilities include material resources – pressure to meet survival necessities like food, clothing, shelter, and safety, lack of money and health insurance, and lack of transportation; and/or communicative structures that stigmatize them and paint them as lazy and incompetent. Structures that can influence outcomes of public health initiatives in sex worker communities include stigmatization and marginalization; limited economic options; limited access to health, social, and legal services; limited access to information and prevention means; gender-related differences and inequalities; sexual exploitation and trafficking; harmful or lack of protective legislation and policies; and exposure to risks associated with lifestyle. Media structures also contribute significantly to foster and further this stigma associated with sex work. For example, the Academy Award–winning documentary *Born into Brothels* on sex workers and their children in Sonagachi, a red-light district in the city of Kolkata in India, paints sex workers as irresponsible mothers who fail to take care of their children (Basu & Dutta, 2011).

In instances such as those of sex workers and the homeless, structures impede their access to organized civil society frameworks that shape their lives (Basu & Dutta, 2008). Their lack of a meaningful say in civil society platforms also means that their concerns and living contexts do not find a voice in the framing of laws and policies that influence health and living. Thus, national and international public health campaigns and policies are formulated by experts without taking into account or seeking to alter structural matrices that influence health behaviors in such spaces.

The culture-centered approach to health communication seeks to foreground these structural factors as realities in the lives of marginalized people, realities that have a profound influence on their health. In doing so, the culture-centered approach situates the creation and reinforcement of structural frameworks in the realm of the political and as hegemonic exercises directed at maintaining the status quo. The aim of such political processes is to ensure that the power to create knowledge and shape health discourses stays outside the reach of subaltern participants, a situation that must be continuously challenged.

Analogous to this logic is the assumption that the subaltern cannot speak, that the subaltern does not have the ability to partake in the construction of the discourse that frames her/his life, and that subaltern spaces are agency-less spaces open to direction and manipulation (Basu, 2011; Dutta, 2008). This logic leads to the mobilization of marginalizing images and discourses, exhuming the subaltern of his/her agency, which serves the political economy of the dominant framework. It ensures that the dominant discourse is able to hold its sway over the knowledge-creation enterprise and over spaces at the margins. The culture-centered approach takes a cue from Subaltern Studies scholarship and attempts to invert this logic. It reframes the notion that the subaltern is not able to speak to one that says that the subaltern is not able to speak in a way that is considered meaningful enough (in terms of codes and guidelines of meaningfulness set by the dominant discourse) to be accommodated in the dominant discursive framework (Beverly, 2004).

Essential to the philosophy of the culture-centered approach is the argument that the subaltern can and does speak but that his voice is confined to the periphery of the modernist discursive paradigm because of mainstream cultural formulations that depict such voices as non-existent or inadequate and the consequent structural conditions that continue to perpetuate the marginalization of these voices. It questions the political motive behind the marginalization of subaltern voices and theorizes that such a move serves to maintain power relations in the archaeology of knowledge and to protect knowledge positions that help to justify the location of subalterns at the margins of health-care systems. The culture-centered approach highlights the participation and voices of community members in the construction of health meanings. It centralizes organic participation and highlights the recognition and respect for subaltern agency.

Agency refers to the capacity of human beings to engage with structures that encompass their lives, to make meanings through this engagement, scripting texts of engagement with the structures, living within these structures and, at the same time, creating discursive openings to transform these structures. Dutta (2008) locates agency at its interaction with culture and structure and notes that the human capability to devise communication strategies by making sense of the structures defining one's life helps to connect to the roots of a culture. Agency documents pathways that cultural members forge and follow to conduct their lives. Simultaneously, the agency that resides in subaltern spaces creates avenues for cultural participants to use the resources at their disposal to change and transform structures that impede their ability to lead healthy lives (Dutta, 2008). By highlighting meanings that emerge from within participant spaces, the culture-centered approach asks questions such as, *How do subaltern communities interpret structures within which they live their lives? How do they respond to and resist such structures and frame health meanings and discourses?*

Note that the focus of the culture-centered approach is not on "empowering" the subaltern subjects from outside, as this very stance once again assumes the implied expertise of the researcher and strips the subaltern participant of his agency. In the culture-centered approach, the emphasis is not on creating skills such that community members can be empowered through the campaign after being taught the necessary interpersonal communication skills (see, e.g., Storey & Jacobson, 2003). Rather, the emphasis is on understanding existing forms of participation and resistance in communities that have traditionally been treated as devoid of agency (Dutta-Bergman, 2004a; Dutta, 2008). Inherent here is the idea that subaltern communities exercise their will in challenging structures through their day-to-day practices (Bhadra, 1997). It is the task of public health scholars and practitioners to find ways to listen to such stories of participation and resistance and be responsive to them. The culture-centered approach begins with the understanding that real consciousness, as opposed to false consciousness that resides in subaltern spaces, engenders participation in these marginalized spaces that typically have been conceptualized as recipients of public health interventions.

Agency as resistance

Drawing from Subaltern Studies (Guha & Spivak, 1988), the culture-centered approach articulates the ways in which subaltern groups resist structural constraints and challenge existing cultural and contextual frames. The emphasis is on resistance as a communicative act that challenges the dominant structures and seeks to transform them (Basu & Dutta, 2008; Dutta, 2008, 2011, 2013). The centers of power that participate in the marginalization of the subaltern classes are interrogated, and opportunities are sought for their transformation. This approach to health promotion seeks answers to questions such as the following:

- How do individuals, groups, and communities participate in communication in order to critique and transform the dominant social system that contributes to their marginalization?
- What discursive openings do marginalized communities create for articulating avenues for social change in order to secure access to structures that will facilitate healthy living contexts? For instance, in the case of sex workers, what are the ways in which communities create cultural meanings that resist stigmatizing messages that continue to justify their existence at the margins and lack of access to health resources?

"Resistance" refers to those communicative processes and messages that directly challenge the structures that constrain the life experiences of subaltern groups with the goal of changing these structures (Haynes & Prakash, 1992). As a communicative act in the context of health-promotion practices, resistance needs to be theorized along a spectrum, including challenges to the dominant discursive constructions; the ownership of agency in determining community-relevant solutions; and the mobilization of resources to create alternative communicative frameworks, structural resources, and overt confrontational practices that seek to challenge and fight violence that is imposed on subaltern spaces. The culture-centered approach constructs resistance as a continually transformative communicative process that emerges and evolves in relationship to structure (Pal & Dutta, 2008). Dominance and hegemony are situated in a dialectical relationship with each other, founding and confounding each other through consistently reconfigurative processes. Resistance in the context of public health communication is both an everyday practice enacted through day-to-day actions that challenge the dominant structures, and a practice of organizing and mobilizing for more overt forms of communication directed toward challenging structures (Haynes & Prakash, 1992).

For example, at the micro level, resistance is played out in the individual choices that community members make in response to their marginalization and as a challenge to dominant epistemic foundations in health communication. This might involve non-compliance with health recommendations offered by the dominant biomedical system as was seen in the "natives'" resistance to immunization efforts of the British in pre-independence India (Arnold, 1993). Or in the framing of health and disease as a function, cause, and effect of disruption in nature and natural processes as opposed to modernist constructions in the realm of pathogens, preventions, and cures, evident among Santali communities (Dutta-Bergman, 2004a, 2004b). At the macro-level, resistance might comprise challenging the broader communicative frameworks that create, shape, and reify marginalization. This might involve participating in mainstream political and social processes that advocate, design, and implement norms, rules, and laws – political parties, non-governmental organizations, and/or media platforms (Dutta-Bergman, 2004a). An example of this is the formation of trade unions and cultural organizations by sex workers in Sonagachi. Sex workers here have mobilized community members to form to a non-governmental organization (NGO) called the Durbar Mahila Samanwyay Committee (DMSC) that fights for their rights as workers. The DMSC is also engaged in planning, designing, implementing, and evaluating an HIV/AIDS campaign within the community, besides organizing sex workers in their fight against structural and physical violence. Basu and Dutta (2008, 2009, 2013) document the ways in which resistance is played out in sex worker spaces in relationship to structures that surround the health experiences of community members. Supporting the notion of subaltern agency, participant narratives that emerge from two sex worker communities in Kolkata point to the variety of ways in which members of a marginalized culture find opportunities to voice concerns and work toward empowerment and change.

Empowerment, in this context, is thought of as a communicative process through which individuals and groups in marginalized spaces express themselves and articulate their needs. Empowerment is seen as a process where the community members are out of touch with communication avenues that would enable them to articulate their needs. This is in contrast to the top-down form of empowerment dominating much of the current scholarship on participatory public health programs, which is based on the "hallowed pretext that one (usually all-knowing academics) can empower another (the disenfranchised)" (C. Airhihenbuwa, 2007, p. 128), and which focuses on "celebrated linear behavior theories and models to chart how 'these unfortunate souls' can be 'empowered' to overcome the forces that have circumscribed their potential for 'normal well-being'" (p. 127). In their study of sex work and health, Basu and Dutta (2008) state that sex worker narratives point to ways in which empowerment materializes from within in the way they are able to articulate and implement structures that cater to their fundamental health needs (such as setting up a micro-credit organization). In this sense, agency and consciousness are not elements that are introduced into a marginalized community by outsiders (read public health practitioners) but are intrinsic to the existence of structural oppressions within social systems.

Participation is the essence of the communicative act of resistance and acts as an avenue for participant-driven social change. Subaltern participation in the articulation of their own health problems is considered a step toward achieving meaningful change (Guha, 1997; Guha & Spivak, 1988). According to the culture-centered approach, subaltern participants are indeed able to take stock of the structures that define their lives and limit possibilities of good health; engage with these structures to locate their health needs; and plan, design, implement, and evaluate strategies that help them achieve their desired health goals. In doing so, the culture-centered approach centralizes the voices of subaltern communities, brought forth through the conversations between the researcher and the community participants. Dutta-Bergman (2004a) states that the culture-centered approach emphasizes dialogue, listening, and mutual understanding, locating the agency for examining health practices in the culture being studied, not in the researcher and the institutional practices that inform his research. It is through this dialogic participatory agenda that local cultural articulations on health are instituted into the dominant discursive space.

In the culture-centered approach then, health problems are identified by participants in the cultural space; participants engage with available structural resources and determine plans of action (Dutta-Bergman, 2004a, 2004b; Dutta, 2008). The culture-centered approach centralizes the narratives that emerge from these participatory acts in marginalized spaces and introduces them into discursive frameworks that have systematically chosen to erase them through one-way models built upon the assumed expertise of the public health scholar/practitioner. These narratives act as resistive scripts as they not only articulate subaltern agency, but also seek to subvert the dominant narratives on what constitutes health and illness.

The public health scholar's participation in co-creating the narratives and acts of resistance to health initiatives formulated in the dominant discursive space speak to notions of solidarity, of friendship with spaces around the world that have been consistently categorized as deficient and in need to be hidden. So, instead of imposing health interventions on marginalized communities, the effort is to understand how health is enacted in these spaces, to listen to the narratives that come out of spaces as members engage with their limited resources to make meanings of health and lives, and to introduce the co-created scripts into those mainstream discursive structures that have so long buried them. In other words, the co-constructive process of meaning creation that the culture-centered approach to health communication emphasizes creates spaces for marginalized people to frame their own discourses on health, discourses that are often situated as resistances to the dominant public health discourse.

Forms of resistance

In this section, we will work through various forms of resistance and demonstrate through these forms the interplays of culture, structure, and agency in inverting the dominant articulations of public health efforts. We present narratives of resistance from several subaltern spaces (recorded in our research projects across West Bengal, India, and Singapore) into discursive sites of public health communication. They appear as communicative inversions, rendering impure the ontologies of public health interventions and making visible the otherwise hidden assumptions that constitute these interventions. Resistance as reflected in this section is constituted in everyday acts of meaning making on health and illness. Simultaneously, resistance is enacted through communication as sharing and through collective participation in mobilizing alternative frameworks of transformation.

Resistance as memory

Resistance is constituted in the remembering of public health communication efforts that have been framed in dominant discourses as instruments of modernity. Discourses of modernity and the success of top-down interventions are interrupted by the voices of the subaltern, re-reading the scripts of public health interventions in inverse. The act of remembering is the telling of another story, a story that ruptures, bringing forth voices of affect that draw up from the body stories in reverse.

Jamuna remembers the time that she was cheated into having an operation (she is referring to a tubectomy campaign that was carried out across the slums in her area). She remembers how she went into the check-up thinking it was going to be a general physical examination, looking forward to earning the money that would help feed her family. The rains continued incessantly that monsoon season. Many days had gone by, and there was no money for the family. So when she heard about the health camp being conducted at the *Moidaan* (a large field where camps and circuses are usually held), she was excited. The 50 rupees she would make at the end of the day was money for one or two days' food, depending upon how she used the money. The camp was a set of white tents spread all over the field. When she walked in, a few of the *didis* (referring to urban middle class educated women, signifying a difference in power, a difference in where one belongs in a hierarchy) hurriedly took her aside and had her sign on a form. She did not know what was in the form, but she signed it anyways. Jamuna was quickly moved to a makeshift operation table, the doctor saying that she was going to do a surgery that would help her feel better. Jamuna does not recall what happened after that, tears streaming down her eyes. She recalls waking up with pain. The *didis* gave her a banana and an egg, and handed her the 50 rupees note. She recounts how after many days she realized that her tubes had been tied. She says she is filled with rage at this memory. This act of remembering is also an act of acknowledging the deception and mistreatment she attaches to middle class *babus* and *didis*. She says that the *bhadralok* (referring to middle class Bengalis who often occupy the professional positions of health workers, public health staff, nurses, and doctors) will do anything to sell off the poor.

Jamuna's memory stands in resistance to the dominant narratives of public health communication written by the middle classes that she is suspicious of. Her suspicion of the intent and credibility of the middle classes is deeply rooted in her body and in her experience of deception. Her depiction of communication as deception attends to the misleading tools of the dominant structures of public health communication efforts, which in an attempt to persuade, deploy various misleading strategies. She is skeptical of persuasion because persuasion for her is deception. Her recollection of how she was not informed about what was going to happen, what was done to her body, and what would be the consequences to her resist the dominant narrative of the "*Hum do, hamare do*" (We two, our two) campaign. The glittery posters of the campaign with images of a happy family of four (father, mother, boy, and girl) are disrupted by Jamuna's recollection of the materiality of violence marked on her body. The stories of pain, loss, and unexplained physical symptoms interrupt the monolithic narratives of public health communication built on the framework of persuasion and social marketing.

When remembering her bodily symptoms since the surgery, Jamuna questions the violence of public health that exploited her body by deceiving her. She shares that the *babus* and *didis* made money from doing the surgery and left her bereft. She shares that her ability to have a child was stolen from her for 50 rupees, and voices that this is the price of the life of the poor in India. Jamuna's resistance disrupts the narratives of public health communication as directed at improving the health and well-being of the poor, instead offering an alternative anchor for interpreting public health interventions. Her narration interrupts the dominant discourse by depicting the ways in which the portrayal of the poor as a silent body works to enact violence. She shares that the *babus* did not even think of her as a human being, and that is why they could carry out the violence on her body. Public health as a form of violence stands in as a reminder of the instruments of the state, public workers, and public agencies in silencing the voices of the poor. Jamuna's narrative is a reminder, an invitation to recollect the stories of erasure and invasion constituted in public health communication interventions.

Resistance as talk

Through everyday conversations with each other, members of subaltern communities interrogate the narratives circulated in the dominant structures of public health communication efforts. Relationships of trust with one another offer resistive frameworks for interrogating the narratives of progress and well-being depicted in public health communication materials. Talk is a resource of resistance and sustenance. Through talk, participants co-create networks of information sharing that can challenge the top-down information being disseminated by public health campaigns. Talk thus becomes a form of fact-checking, as a way for assessing the trustworthiness of the information received. Talk also becomes a way of sharing with others one's own experiences. This is especially essential to public health communication efforts that are directed by a dominant agenda seeking to undermine the sovereignty of the community.

Let us, for instance, listen to the voice of Jamuna. After going through her violent experience with a deceptive public health intervention, Jamuna talks to the other women in her family so they do not go through similar experiences. In conversing with other women in her interpersonal networks, she makes sure that the story of violence she experienced is shared. She also makes sure to talk to other women in her network about strategies of deciphering the agendas of a health-care worker or a health team. For instance, one of the things she shares is to not be rushed into having to make a decision on the spot. Recalling her experience, she shares how she was treated like cattle and did not really have any opportunities to ask any questions. Therefore, she teaches "question asking" as an important strategy to her peers and family members. She tells others: "Always ask questions. Don't just go with what the *babus* say. And if your question is not answered, then walk away." She shares how she will not make a decision without being given greater depth and detail on a topic in future. Through her talks with other women, she shares these strategies of returning the gaze on public health communication efforts.

On a similar note, an advisory board of transgender sex workers who have come together to put together a culture-centered project rooted in their lived experiences discuss public health communication efforts that usually target them, and share how they use strategies of talking to one another in challenging the stigmatizing messages they receive from mainstream health campaigns. Savitri, a 26-year-old Indian sex worker, remembers the previous campaign she had participated in. She discusses the ways in which the campaign treated her as a body that is a site of HIV risk. She felt humiliated and stripped of her dignity. In resisting the depiction of the transgender community in the campaign, Savitri talked about the campaign and its messages with other transgender sex workers, actively decoding the messages to take the sting away from the messages.

Resistance as everyday acts

Resistance is constituted in the everyday negotiations of public health communication interventions that are targeted at communities at the margins. Mia shares how as a sex worker, she has this perennial feeling of being a target, of being under a panopticon, having been fixed as high risk. Her body is marked as a site of intervention, having been identified as a source of disease. Mia shares how she resists HIV/AIDS interventions targeted at her by refusing to talk to community peer leaders. She shares how often she will walk away. In other instances, when there is some monetary promise attached, she will participate, but instead of being a passive listener, she uses the opportunities of interactions with peer leaders for an established HIV/AIDS campaign to draw attention to the stigmas they circulate through the messages they give out. She recalls her experience of an interaction with a peer leader. When the peer leader asked her some questions about her sexual behavior, rather than simply responding to the yes/no questions, Mia began a conversation with the peer leader. She asked more questions in return, asking the peer leader to reflect on her own assumptions and biases. For instance, when the peer leader asked her about the how frequently she asked her clients to use a condom, Mia asked the peer leader why she was instead not interviewing clients, as she would then get a better idea. Noting that she could not potentially understand what's going on in the client's head, Mia took the opportunity to educate the peer leader that HIV prevention work is much more likely to be effective when taking clients into account and bringing them into the conversation. These everyday acts of resistance she hoped would change how campaigns are thought of and carried out.

In another example of resistance, Jonardon shared how he avoided the public health workers whenever they came for rounds to his village. He shared that he would mostly just disappear whenever she saw the *didimonis* (referring to the public health workers, mostly women who came to the village, usually dressed in white saris with blue border) around the village. When asked why he disappeared, he shared that he usually did not see any value to the papers the *didis* handed out. The *didis*, he noted were nowhere to be seen when a health need arises in the family, and only come to give out information that he finds of no use. Because the time during the day is valuable, he says that he would rather use the time to work the fields and/or earn money as a day laborer. Rearticulating his time and labor as integral to his everyday struggle, Jonardon resisted the extraction of the unpaid labor of participants in public health efforts that served the agendas of the dominant sections of society. In this, the everyday act of simply avoiding public health workers also emerges as a site for rearticulating labor.

Everyday acts of resistance are also shared in stories of deliberate misrepresentation when being asked a question. Sharon, a mother of three, earning 980 USD per month from her job as a waitress, shares how she does not exactly share the truth when responding to public health workers carrying out interventions. She shares how when stopped by a red booth (promoting heart health) and being promised 14 USD for completing a survey and listening to a small talk, she shares inaccurate information so she can earn the money and yet not have to disclose personal health details. She says that the person asking the question would ask personal questions like how much salt she eats, how much rice she eats, and how many times she exercises. Most of this information she cannot recall. Other information she knows will portray her poorly, and that would make her feel bad about herself. She copes with this potential sense of feeling bad by deliberately sharing incorrect information that would portray her as being healthy. This strategy of resistance is also a strategy for coping with her sense of identity. Through her sharing of inaccurate information, Sharon recrafts an everyday strategy of resisting the gaze and surveillance of public health campaigns.

In the various everyday acts of resistance, public health as an instrument of the dominant sector is challenged. Noting the ways in which public health efforts serve the agendas and goals of those in power, those at the margins depict strategies for inverting the dominant articulations of experts. Everyday forms of negotiation point toward strategies of inverting the otherwise one-way flow of communication and information from experts to target communities at the margins. Resistance is in these narratives as part of everyday life, constituted in everyday acts of interrogating the dominant power structures and the dominant narratives of public health. Resistance is also reiterated in the everyday acts of resisting the surveillance and scripting carried out by public health programs.

Resistance as collective participation

Resistance in subaltern contexts emerges into the mainstream through collective narratives. Subaltern struggles emerge at specific points and sites of articulation as entry points to alternative imaginations. The coming together as a collective is constituted around contingent and flexible identities that are stitched together into a collective to articulate an agenda for change. These identities, however, are continually in flux. Simultaneously evident in the subaltern narratives of resistance are the structures that erase these voices; in negotiating these structures, subaltern communities craft out impermanent identities that appear in discourses and simultaneously disappear. Subalternity as erasure from discursive spaces and sites of articulation is salient across various culture-centered projects, and yet a form of strategically essentialist position is adopted by subaltern communities to appear into hegemony as collectives, however briefly, to make claims to rights of representation and recognition in discourses of health and well-being. The transitive nature of these collectives also then suggests that the enacted identities are fragile, often disappearing after the articulations have been made and positions have been crafted out in the mainstream.

One of our culture-centered collaborations with Santali communities in the Jangalmahal area of West Bengal, India, often negotiates these transitive identities as specific claims are made at discursive sites. When, for instance, the state introduced a public health campaign on promoting safe drinking water targeting the villages, community members came together as a collective to question the value of a campaign sending out the message in leaflets and making announcements on speakers traveling on rickshaws. Villagers collected together in an advisory board meeting and came up with the idea that they wanted to challenge the strategy of information dissemination through giving out leaflets and making announcements. Organizing a petition across the village, they collected signatures instead to use the opportunity to pressure the block development officer to build a clean drinking water source in the Santali para. The presence of the Santali voices organized in a collective signature campaign challenged the state's narrative of public health promotion and simultaneously used the narrative to develop resources the community needed.

In a culture-centered project with transgender sex workers, we found that the coming together around a collective identity was an entry point to changing the typical erasure of voices in public health communication efforts. Laila, a transgender sex worker participant in the project that she and her advisory board collaborators labelled as "The Stiletto Project," described the importance of redefining the narratives of public health that portray transgender sex workers as diseased bodies. She describes the difficulties in articulating an identity as a transgender sex worker, constituted amid the various stigmas that emerge from public health campaigns. Sharing how the transgender sex worker community is a target of HIV/AIDS interventions, she described the role of the collective in articulating alternative identities and performances that challenge the monolithic narratives of transgender sex workers as pathological, deviant, and lacking. The work of the collective under the umbrella of "The Stiletto Project" was redefined in terms of overall health and well-being of transgender sex workers, addressing stigmatizing, and developing health information infrastructures on sex reassignment surgery and hormone therapy.

Resistance as collective participation, therefore, inverts the dominant notions and articulations of public health communication efforts. Through collective processes of organizing, communities, whose voices have hitherto been erased from public health discourses, directly challenge the discourses, offering alternative interpretations and discursive constructions. The dominant discourses of public health communication that construct targeted communities as passive and devoid of agency are disrupted through the collective participation of subaltern communities in processes of change.

Redefining public health communication

The forms of resistance voiced in this chapter point toward the classed, gendered, caste-based oppressions that are written into the dominant frameworks of public health communication. These voices of resistance suggest that public health communication is written in a script of violence, pointing to the various forms of violence that are written into the interventions, often tied to the depiction of communities as targets. The human dignity and agentic capacities of communities are stolen from them in the depiction of them as target audiences of campaigns designed by bourgeoisie experts occupying the status quo. As tools of the structure, traditional domains of public health communication efforts continue to reify dominant ideas of subaltern communities as devoid of agency. The erasure of subaltern agency then becomes the justification for top-down interventions. Having foreclosed the possibilities of subaltern voices, the expert administrator and public health planner emerge at discursive sites as designers, evaluators, and commentators on public health interventions. Essential to the violence of public health communication is the unquestioned narrative of doing good, rooted in the mission-like imperial orientation of the campaign planner. Resistance offers a framework for redefining public health communication, rooting public health communication in the lived experiences of communities in the global South, and co-creating invitational spaces for subaltern voices to render impure the dominant agendas of public health. Through subaltern participation in public health decision-making processes and in infrastructures of communication, entry points are reimagined for public health as social justice.

Editor commentary

Mohan Dutta and Ambar Basu have offered a foundation upon which to explore, to think through, resistance to public health efforts in their perspective of *culture-centered* approaches. Distinct from *culturally sensitive* approaches, which are developed by outside experts in recognition of and with sensitivity toward local context, the culture-centered approach, as expressed in this chapter, centralizes participation, engagement, and collaboration with target populations, often the subaltern or marginalized communities. Through these often slow and long-term engagements, agency is fostered. While agency may result in resistance to public health structures, allowing space for the existence or development of agency is one strategy to accommodate successful collaboration. In addition, the authors identify and explore different forms of resistance, including the following:

- Resistance as memory
- Resistance as talk
- Resistance as everyday acts, including avoidance, passivity, and non-compliance
- Resistance as collective participation, an area further explored in Chapter 8

References

Airhihenbuwa, C. (2007). *Healing Our Differences: The Crisis of Global Health and the Politics of Identity*. Lanham, MD: Rowman & Littlefield.

Airhihenbuwa, C., & Obregon, R. (2000). A critical assessment of theories/models used in health communication for HIV/AIDS. *Journal of Health Communication, 5*(Suppl1), 5–15.

Airhihenbuwa, C. O. (1995). *Health and Culture: Beyond the Western Paradigm*. Thousand Oaks, CA: Sage.

Arnold, D. (1993). *Colonizing the Body: State Medicine and Epidemic Disease in Nineteenth-Century India*. Berkeley: University of California Press.

Basu, A. (2011). HIV/AIDS and subaltern autonomous rationality: A call to re-center health communication in marginalized sex worker spaces. *Communication Monographs, 78*(3), 391–408.

Basu, A., & Dutta, M. J. (2008). Participatory change in a campaign led by sex workers: Connecting resistance to action-oriented agency. *Qualitative Health Research, 18*(1), 106–119.

Basu, A., & Dutta, M. J. (2009). Sex workers and HIV/AIDS: Analyzing participatory culture-centered health communication strategies. *Human Communication Research, 35*, 86–114.

Basu, A., & Dutta, M. J. (2011). 'We are mothers first': Localocentric articulation of sex worker identity as a keyword in HIV/AIDS communication. *Women & Health, 51*(2), 106–123.

Basu, A., & Dutta, M. J. (2013). Health and sex work: Structures as narrative nodes. In A. Mishra & S. Chatterjee (Eds.), *Narratives of Health and Illness: Readings from Asia*. Delhi: Orient Blackswan.

Beverly, J. (2004). *Subalternity and Representation: Arguments in Cultural Theory*. Durham, NC: Duke University Press.

Bhadra, G. (1997). The mentality of the subaltern. In R. Guha (Ed.), *A Subaltern Studies Reader, 1986–1995* (pp. 63–99). Minneapolis, MN: University of Minnesota Press.

Dutta, M. J. (2008). *Communicating Health: A Culture-Centered Approach*. Cambridge, UK: Polity.

Dutta, M. J. (2011). *Communicating Social Change: Structure, Culture, and Agency*. New York, NY: Taylor & Francis.

Dutta, M. J. (2013). *Voices of Resistance*. West Lafayette, IN: Purdue University Press.

Dutta-Bergman, M. J. (2004a). Poverty, structural barriers, and health: A Santali narrative of health communication. *Qualitative Health Research, 14*(8), 1107–1122.

Dutta-Bergman, M. J. (2004b). The unheard voice of Santalis: Communicating about health from the margins of India. *Communication Theory, 14*(3), 237–263.

Dutta-Bergman, M. J. (2005). Theory and practice in health communication campaigns: A critical interrogation. *Health Communication, 182*, 103–122.

Fanon, F. (1968). *The Wretched of the Earth*. New York: Grove Press.

Ford, A., & Yep, G. (2003). Working along the margins: Developing community-based strategies for communication about health with marginalized groups. In T. Thompson, A. Dorsey, K. Miller, & R. Parrott (Eds.), *Handbook of Health Communication* (pp. 241–262). Mahwah, NJ: Erlbaum.

Foss, S.K., & Griffin, C.L. (1995). Beyond persuasion: A proposal for an invitational rhetoric. *Communication Monographs, 62*, 2–18.

Foucault, M. (1984). The body of the condemned. In P. Rabinow (Ed.), *The Foucault Reader* (pp. 51–75). New York: Pantheon.

Geertz, C. (1973). Thick description: Toward an interpretive theory of culture. In C. Geertz (Ed.), *The Interpretation of cultures* (pp. 3–30). London: Hutchinson.

Guha, R. (1997). Introduction. In R. Guha (Ed.), *A Subaltern Studies Reader* (pp. ix–xii). Minneapolis, MN: University of Minnesota Press.

Guha, R., & Spivak, G. (Eds.). (1988). *Selected Subaltern Studies.* New Delhi: Oxford University Press.

Haynes, D., & Prakash, G. (1992). Introduction: The entanglement of power and resistance. In D. Haynes & G. Prakash (Eds.), *Contesting Power: Resistance and Everyday Social Relations in South Asia* (pp. 1–22). Berkeley: University of California Press.

Helman, C. (1986). *Culture, Health and Illness.* Bristol, UK: Wright.

Lupton, D. (1994). Toward the development of critical health communication praxis. *Health Communication, 6,* 55–67.

Lupton, D. (2003). *Medicine as Culture.* Thousand Oaks, CA: Sage.

Nandy, A. (1988). Modern medicine and its nonmodern critics: A study in discourse. In A. Nandy (Ed.), *The Savage Freud and Other Possible Essays on Possible and Retrievable Selves* (pp. 145–195). Princeton, NJ: Princeton University Press.

Pal, M., & Dutta, M. J. (2008). Theorizing resistance in a global context: processes, strategies and tactics in communication scholarship. In C. Beck (Ed.), *Communication Yearbook* (Vol. 32, pp. 41–87). New York: Routledge.

Storey, D., & Jacobson, T. (2003). Entertainment-education and participation: Applying Habermas to a population program in Nepal. In A. Singhal, M. Cody, E. Rogers, & M. Sabido (Eds.), *Entertainment-Education and Social Change: History, Research, and Practice* (pp. 417–434). Mahwah, NJ: Lawrence Erlbaum.

WHO (1948). About: World Health Organization. Retrieved from http://www.who.int/about/definition/en/print.html

Wilkins, K., & Mody, B. (2001). Reshaping development communication: Developing communication and communicating development. *Communication Theory, 11*(4), 385–396.

3

"PROTECTING LIFE"

The Case of Texas Legislation and Resistances to Gardasil, the HPV Vaccine

Samantha D. Gottlieb

The Texas order

In early February 2007, Texas governor and future presidential candidate Rick Perry issued what would be a contentious executive order, RP 65. Bypassing the Texas legislatures' discussions of similar policies (H.B. 215, 2007; S.B. 110, 2007), RP 65 required sixth-grade girls in Texas public schools receive the newly approved human papillomavirus (HPV) vaccine, Gardasil (Blumenthal, 2007; Perry, 2007). Gardasil targets HPV, the most common sexually transmitted infection (STI), which has been linked to cervical cancer. The Federal Drug Administration (FDA) approved its use in June 2006 for 9–26-year-old females; as for other childhood vaccines, a number of state legislatures introduced legislation to require Gardasil. Perry articulated his motivations:

> Never before have we had an opportunity to prevent cancer with a simple vaccine. While I understand the concerns expressed by some, *I stand firmly on the side of protecting life*. The HPV vaccine *does not promote sex*, it *protects women's health*. In the past, young women who have abstained from sex until marriage have contracted HPV from their husbands and faced the difficult task of defeating cervical cancer. This vaccine prevents that from happening.
>
> Providing *the HPV vaccine doesn't promote sexual promiscuity* anymore [sic] than providing the Hepatitis B vaccine promotes drug use. If the medical community developed a vaccine for lung cancer, would the same critics oppose it claiming it would encourage smoking?
>
> Finally, parents need to know that they have the final decision about whether or not their daughter is vaccinated. *I am a strong believer in protecting parental rights*, which is why this executive order allows them *to opt out*. (Perry, cited in Anonymous, 2007, italics added)

In this brief statement, Perry raised fraught political issues in the U.S.: parents' rights, vaccine policies, and adolescent (especially female) sexualities. Perry's pro-life invocation to justify his order, requiring parents to submit their daughters to this new medical technology, draws attention to the biopolitical nature of his actions.

Biopolitics, a concept developed by Foucault, is a distinctly historical theory, incorporating the specificity of time and place, the economics, structures, and politics of a particular moment. Drawing on classical theories of sovereignty, which allowed rulers "the right over life and death" (Foucault & Ewald, 2003, p. 240), Foucault sees power as a dynamic process throughout history. Contemporary social scientists continue to expand how biopower and biopolitics function. Rabinow and Rose emphasize that Foucault uses "'biopolitics' to embrace all the specific strategies and contestations over problematizations of collective human vitality, morbidity and mortality" (2003, p. 197). Biopower operates through multiple institutions, *not just* sovereign states, and a "unified governmental discourse" does not exist (Leach & Fairhead, 2007, p. 38).

One manifestation of biopower is through "biomedicalization," a term referring to the technosciences and the evolving "multisited, multidirectional processes" of medicalization (Clarke, Shim, Mamo, & Fosket, 2003, p. 162).[1] Biopolitics and biomedicalization are part of biopower's pervasive reaches. Perry's statement references the range of human existence: life to illness to (the threat of) death. Through executive privilege, Perry tried, and ultimately failed, to set the terms of vaccinating young female bodies. The public's reactions to the order came swiftly after the RP 65 announcement. They took a variety of forms, but they all deployed legal or policy strategies to resist the governor's dictum. I explore these responses to Perry as resistances, not refusals, to capture their form of collective action, rather than individual stances (Hobson-West, 2003; Streefland, Chowdhury, & Ramos-Jimenez, 1999). Yet, although these strategies may be read as resistances, I will contend an alternative interpretation – as participation in biopower's multiplicity.

HPV vaccine – limitations and utility

The FDA's June 2006 approval for Gardasil occurred only six months after Merck's initial submission to the national regulatory agency (Harris, 2006b). Gardasil's potential cervical cancer mortality reduction motivated the agency to fast track its review. Among the hundred types of HPV, about 40 types are sexually transmitted (Muñoz, Castellsagué, de González, & Gissmann, 2006). Of the sexually transmitted types of HPV, some produce genital warts, while others can develop into cancers. Almost all cases of cervical cancer start with HPV, but infection with cancerous HPV does not *necessarily* lead to cancer. Many people never know they are infected, as HPV infections often clear on their own. Although HPV is very common, the associated cancers are less so. HPV can lead to anal, penile, and oral cancers, but these receive significantly less discussion in the media.

Cervical cancer is preventable when caught early through regular gynecological screening, but it remains a leading cause of death for women globally (Jemal, Bray, Center, Ferlay, Ward, & Forman, 2011). There is no test for HPV in men, even though both men and women can be infected through sexual contact. Cervical cancer kills around 4,000 U.S. women a year. This number has not increased for more than two decades (Singh, 2012), largely due to the Pap smear's institutionalization, which facilitates treating women before cancer progresses.[2] Women in countries with limited access to screening suffer from much higher cervical cancer mortality, a leading cause of death for women in less industrialized countries (P. Adams, 2012). Although most U.S. women receive Pap smears, prior to Gardasil's market debut, few women were aware of HPV or its association with cervical cancer (Baer, Allen, & Braun, 2000; D'Urso, Thompson-Robinson, & Chandler, 2007; Friedman & Shepeard, 2007; Klug, Hukelmann, & Blettner, 2008). The persistent 4,000 U.S. cervical cancer deaths likely reflect limitations that Gardasil cannot address, such as cost, time, or lack of awareness that affect women's access to care. It is unclear how much impact the HPV vaccines will have on cervical cancer mortality in the U.S., when those at risk for cervical cancer mortality may have attributes or access issues unrelated to vaccination uptake.

When Perry issued his executive order, Gardasil was a quadrivalent vaccine, offering protection against HPV 16 and 18, associated with cervical cancer, and HPV 6 and 11, which can cause genital warts. In 2006–2007, Gardasil was the most expensive vaccine on the market, costing nearly $400 for the full series (Harris, 2006a; Johnson, 2007). Its recipients must receive a three-shot series over specific intervals for vaccine efficacy. Approved in December 2014, Gardasil's newer version, protects against nine types of HPV. In this chapter, I refer to Gardasil's quadrivalent version. Cervarix, manufactured by Merck's competitor, GlaxoSmithKline, received FDA approval in 2009; unlike Gardasil, Cervarix protects against only HPV 16 and 18. Although there are now two HPV vaccines, in the first years after Gardasil's approval during preliminary state legislatures' debates, HPV vaccine policies were brand-specific. Further, Gardasil was *the only* female-specific vaccine, receiving reimbursement by insurance companies and subsidized by state agencies.

Novel tools may promise radical reconfiguring of treatment, but in practice such technologies join preexisting conceptions and categories. "New medical technologies are good to think with" (Wynn & Trussell, 2006, p. 297), for they reveal how medicine and science extend beyond the clinic, engaging with social and cultural values to which the technologies may contribute (Parthasarathy, 2005). New technologies' implications are rarely predictable. Engaging actors, resources, knowledge, and power (Lehoux & Blume, 2000), vaccines inform global health and economic policies, and they elicit parents' personal decisions for their children. Positioned by Merck and public health proponents as a critical shift in women's health prevention,[3] Gardasil became enmeshed in U.S. debates about general vaccine practices and how public officials, clinicians, and parents negotiate health decisions. Perry's order and its subsequent reactions demonstrate that, "scientific knowledge . . . both embeds and is embedded in social practices, identities, norms, conventions, discourses, instruments and institutions" (Jasanoff, 2004, p. 3). Gardasil's contestations were almost never about scientific concerns but instead moral and political debates about power, bodies, and authority.

Prior to Gardasil's approval, women's health advocates worried that conservative political bias would delay its approval (Pollitt, 2005); another women's health technology, over-the-counter emergency contraception, Plan B, had recently received protracted FDA approval due to politicized, and not scientific, concerns about its acceptability (Wynn & Trussell, 2006). Merck's pre- and post-licensure advertisements positioned Gardasil as the *cervical cancer* vaccine, rather than as an STI vaccine (Gottlieb, 2013; Mamo & Epstein, 2014). In the U.S., before FDA licensure, companies cannot market pharmaceutical products' names explicitly. Merck primed Gardasil's potential market for the vaccine's arrival, with an ambiguous television and print campaign encouraging women to "Tell Someone." In two television advertisements, women expressed surprise that cervical cancer was "caused by a virus," and although they mentioned HPV, the ads neither acknowledged HPV's sexual transmission nor men (Tell Someone, 2006).

Merck's initial Gardasil FDA submission included data for boys and girls (FDA, 2006), but the FDA found the male data lacking.[4] In television and print ads, men's absence and the highly gendered representations of female camaraderie suggest that Merck never expected to receive male approval its first round of review (Gottlieb, forthcoming; Thompson, 2010). The FDA would not approve Gardasil's genital warts indication for boys until late 2009, and Gardasil's male anal cancer indication did not receive approval until December 2010 (FDA, 2009, 2010). Whether by design, or by circumstances, Gardasil's availability and its related debates centered on female bodies.

United States vaccine policy and debates

For more than a century, immunization has been a widespread medical and public health practice in the United States. To maximize the number vaccinated (Streefland et al., 1999), state policies, influenced by federal policy recommendations, have linked vaccination to school entry. As compulsory school-based education became common in the 19th century, public health officials used school attendance for increasing vaccination rates. Massachusetts passed an education-vaccination law in the early 1800s; New York followed shortly thereafter; Indiana, Illinois and Wisconsin all passed such laws by the late 19th century (Hodge, 2002). The immunization-for-school-access model makes vaccination parents' rite of passage, as most U.S. children attend public schools. This has encouraged vaccine uptake, but the conflation of health interventions with educational access also elicits parents' objections. U.S. media often frame parents' objections to vaccines as novel, but parents have used legal action to refuse U.S. vaccine policies for more than a century (Allen, 2007; Colgrove, 2006).

The 1905 lawsuit, *Jacobson v. Massachusetts* challenged whether U.S. states might compel individuals to vaccinate and to deny medical exemptions. The Supreme Court affirmed compulsory vaccination as states' constitutional right to "police powers," but it did not address the school-entry strategy or compulsory childhood vaccines (Colgrove, 2006). *Jacobson* did not result in coercive vaccination measures; rather, the U.S. political culture of "principles of liberty and autonomy" focused on persuasion to encourage vaccine acceptance (Colgrove, 2006, p. 11). The courts first addressed school vaccine requirements explicitly in the 1922 Texas case, *Zucht v. King* (Colgrove, 2006), a lawsuit that upheld cities' rights to issue public health regulations. In the 1970s and 1980s, U.S. vaccine safety lawsuits led to the creation of legal and regulatory bodies to manage claims against pharmaceutical manufacturers, including a special compensation program, the Vaccine Injury Compensation Program (Colgrove, 2006; Harris, 2008; Offit, 2008).[5] The legal model positions parents, policymakers, and vaccine manufacturers as in conflict, but others have suggested that parental vaccine anxieties might be imagined as more complex,

> Boundaries are constantly crossed . . . what can appear as a deep gulf between parental and policy perspectives has emerged. . . . [T]he construction of such polarity is a dynamic process. . . . dichotomies between parental and policy worlds should be seen less as pre-existing than as made and remade through interaction. (Leach & Fairhead, 2007, p. 43)

When parents strategically reframe legislation, they deploy classical biopower mechanisms, becoming active co-creators of policies.

In the year after Gardasil's FDA approval, nearly half the U.S. states considered some form of school entry requirement, but only the state of Virginia and the District of Columbia would pass laws (National Conference of State Legislatures, 2007; Pollack & Saul, 2007). Although public health proponents may view schools and immigration/citizenship transitions as ideal settings in which to implement widespread health measures (see the discussion by Horton and Barker in this volume), there is no reason for schools to prioritize health interventions. Health policies help shape schools into a mechanism of biopower. As Foucault suggests, institutions are

> organized as a multiple, automatic, and anonymous power; for although surveillance rests on individuals, its functioning is that of a network of relations . . . it is the apparatus itself as a whole that produces "power" and distributes individuals in this permanent and continuous field. (Rabinow, 1984, p. 192)

From educators' perspectives, schools represent sites for education, not for enforcement of health or other non-education related laws. But in the "entire political technology of life" institutions give

> rise to infinitesimal surveillances, permanent controls, extremely meticulous orderings of space, indeterminate medical or psychological examinations, to an entire micropower concerned with the body . . . as well to comprehensive measures, statistical assessments, and interventions aimed at the entire social body or at groups taken as a whole. (Donzelot, 1979, p. 267)

Vaccine policies, especially tied to educational institutions, exemplify these embedded forms of social control, absorbed by individuals.

Most parents do vaccinate their children according to the recommended pediatric schedule and school requirements, but unlike most required vaccines, Gardasil does not protect against an airborne contagion inadvertently contracted. Parents reacted to Gardasil state policies because it differs from other school entry vaccines (Mamo & Epstein, 2014). Gardasil is for young adolescents, while most required school vaccines are pediatric, received before starting kindergarten. Adolescent and adult vaccines are increasingly common, but state requirements associated with nascent female sexuality heightened parental concerns. Gardasil's protection against the behaviorally transmitted virus, cast as an "avoidable" infection, concerned those who objected to linking sexuality and schools. Further setting Gardasil apart from the other school requirements, no other vaccine was exclusively for girls, highlighting Gardasil's sex specificity at the time of RP 65.

After the FDA approves new vaccines, the Advisory Committee on Immunization Practices (ACIP) reviews them to evaluate whether the vaccines should be recommended. Recommendations lead to government agencies subsidizing vaccines for lower-income families, under the Vaccines for Children program, and affects private insurance coverage. The ACIP's guidance may trigger state policies that interpret ACIP's endorsement as a template for standardized health practices. Neither state policies nor ACIP recommendations force any individual to receive vaccines. However, Gardasil's ACIP recommendations triggered an unanticipated policy for female immigrants seeking U.S. citizenship. The U.S. Citizenship and Immigration Services,[6] following a 1996 requirement for new citizens to receive all vaccines recommended by ACIP and the Centers for Disease Control (CDC), incorporated Gardasil into its criteria. Yet, because the vaccine was still only approved for women, this placed an undue burden on a particular class of citizen seekers. Immigrant rights' advocates objected to Gardasil's high cost and its target of a non-epidemic infection (Longoria, 2008). Furthermore, females seeking citizenship could not exempt themselves from the vaccine, although no other U.S. citizen was comparably compelled to receive Gardasil for citizenship benefits. A year after the enacted policy and protests from the immigrant rights' communities, the CDC issued a notice removing Gardasil from required citizenship vaccines. The revised criteria required vaccination for infections that risk producing an outbreak, have been eliminated, or are in the process of being eliminated in the U.S. (Haddix, 2009), none of Gardasil's attributes. The CDC implicitly acknowledged that the vaccine criteria for new citizens, intended to prevent airborne communicable diseases, did not match the logic to vaccinate with Gardasil.

Authoritarian control and surveillance have long focused on female bodies, as literal and metaphorical bearers of reproductive potential and future children (Browner & Press, 1996; Martin, 2001; Rapp, 2001) and as imagined volatile and excessive bodies (Grosz, 1994; Kapsalis, 1997). The 'asymmetry' of contraceptives for women and lack of comparable ones for men (Oudshoorn, 2003; Van Kammen, 1999) exemplify gendered biomedical discipline. These bodily management tactics are complicit in capitalist models of opportunity and 'anticipatory regimes' (V. Adams, Murphy, & Clarke, 2009). Perry's order and the parental responses demonstrate Gardasil's confluence of capital interests, political maneuvers, and gendered notions of citizenship. "Girlhood is one site . . . where distinctively anticipatory regimes are at stake . . . 'girlhood' has been identified as a crucial site for the creation of 'human capital'" (V. Adams et al., 2009, p. 235). The future-looking anticipation is more than a temporal projection and is a moral economy (V. Adams et al., 2009) through which institutions strategically govern. Perry labeled his order "pro-life," a term historically linked to an antiabortion stance referring to the fetus's life, not to the pregnant woman's life. Here, pro-life implied an investment in women and girls' longevity and vulnerability. Similarly, the immigration requirement invoked moral and political economies for foreign-born women who needed to affirm their compliance to a standard that not even U.S.-born women needed to meet. RP 65 and the immigrant policy imagined future female bodies for whom disease must be managed, imposing a value on whose bodies were deemed worthy of citizenship and public resources.

Gardasil's FDA approval informed diverse institutions of social and medical control. Vaccine policies hold citizens, and particularly those who seek citizen status, accountable for their health management. Bestowing access to schools or citizenship through vaccination delineates responsible citizens. Refusal or failure to follow these decrees necessarily excludes the (female) individual. The seamless incorporation of one federal agency's recommendations into another institution's standards reveals convoluted logics that shape policy interventions. Tying female citizenship and education access to Gardasil vaccination fits into the pervasiveness of biopower. This mechanism of control includes a "truth discourse" about some essential attributes of human existence, often made by experts or authorities who assert their entitlement to make such claims (Rabinow & Rose, 2006, p. 197). In the case of immigrants seeking citizenship, and during the first three years of Gardasil's female-only approval, the authoritative immigration policy implied foreignness that required sanitization prior to citizenship and classic tropes of unbounded, wild, foreign (often non-white), female bodies.

The Texas and immigration policies framed Gardasil requirements in the name of life and health, terms which biopower invokes to legitimate institutional interventions on a group of people. The policies asserted expertise and paternalist interests in two examples of future citizens – young girls and female immigrants. In Texas, Perry's discourse focused on the sanctity and innocence of female vulnerability: even women who abstain from premarital sex are vulnerable to cervical cancer due to their future spouses' (presumed) promiscuity. Of course, STI exposure can happen at any given sexual encounter. Biopower also prompts individuals to take responsibility for themselves to improve their outcomes through "modes of subjectification" (Rabinow & Rose, 2006, p. 197). Biopower invokes self-care, and failure to comply has institutional and moral consequences. RP 65 opponents defended their objections as a form of moral responsibility and protection of their children.

Strategic institutional responses

Shortly after RP 65, under Jane and John Doe pseudonyms, a group of parents filed a lawsuit. Families and legislators tacked between legal and medical discourses. The lawsuit, although just briefly alluded to in national and local media, focused on the bounds of Perry's executive power (Grissom, 2007). "The families claimed that Perry overstepped his authority . . . and sought to block the use of state funds for buying the vaccine until the dispute is resolved" (Coe, 2007). The lawsuit would not go far because the state legislature overturned RP 65 through H.B. 1098 (2007) and S.B. 438 (2007). The legislative and legal strategies reveal biopower's complexity: Perry issued an executive biomedical policy, and the RP 65 oppositions deployed their own institutionally sanctioned biomedical claims.

In addition to the John and Jane Doe lawsuit, a Texas organization, Parents Requesting Open Vaccine Education (PROVE), agitated against RP 65. The organization's leader invited parents to be outraged by Perry's "issuing an intrusive executive order forcing all of our 11 and 12 year old little girls to be vaccinated against this sexually transmitted virus in order to attend the 6th grade!" (VaccineInfo .net, 2007). Another response came from a coalition "Hands Off Our Kids," which included libertarian, future presidential candidate Ron Paul and notable conservatives (non-Texans) Phyllis Schafly and Bob Barr. This group invoked parental rights, the safety of Gardasil, economic concerns, and "*unwarranted overreaching of executive power*" (Hands Off Our Kids Coalition, 2007, italics added). Texas allows for non-medical vaccine exemptions, like all U.S. states except Mississippi and West Virginia (Blinder, 2015); parents may cite religious or philosophical beliefs that justify their exclusion. The coalition disregarded this opt-out right. Their concerns about privacy alluded to the process to receive a Gardasil exemption, but this was standard for all required vaccines. RP 65's opponents framed Gardasil as an exceptional vaccine to give legitimacy to their interventions.

Two weeks after Perry's order, on February 16, U.S. House Representative Gingrey introduced the "The Parental Right to Decide Protection Act." The proposed bill prohibited federal funds for "mandatory HPV vaccine policies" (H.R. 1153, 2007). In U.S. vaccine policy debates, opponents refer to requirements as "mandates," but this term is misleading, as it implies no alternative to vaccination. There have been no U.S. vaccine mandates since World War I (Schwartz, Caplan, Faden, & Sugarman, 2007). Although inaccurate, resisting a "mandate" heightened the urgency of parents' cause. Gingrey's bill did not explicitly cite RP 65, but referenced Texas: "The Texas Medical Association has stated that although it strongly supports the ability of physicians to provide the HPV vaccine, at this point, it does not support a State mandate" (H.R. 1153, 2007, pp. Sec. 2, 8). Mentioning a state medical association in a federal bill makes little sense, but it served as a warning to other states considering HPV vaccine requirements. Withholding federal support would limit the effectiveness of state initiatives to require vaccination. The funds' restrictions would affect low-income women and children most, as the two groups most dependent on state and federal support to access health care. Although the 2007 Gingrey bill died in the House, it was reintroduced in the 2009–2010 session, and again did not pass, highlighting the interrelated nature of vaccine policies on state and federal levels.

Resistances to RP 65 were not framed through patient-specific identities, but by parents serving as proxies for their children in vaccine decision-making, and thus Texas coalitions took on a biosocial cast. Biopower frames individual citizens as responsible for their well-being; contemporary forms of biopower include patient advocacy groups that absorb these responsibilities and agitate for their "rights (and obligations) to life, health and cure" (Rabinow & Rose, 2006, p. 203). Parents who resisted the Texas order shared a collective identity of parenthood and identified as objectors to government involvement in adolescent sexual health. Biosociality "is intimately entwined with identity politics. It encapsulates a movement from patient to active citizen, facilitated by individuals subscribing to, and utilising biomedical categories" (Dimond, Bartlett, & Lewis, 2015, p. 2). In other health debates, patient activism has actively shaped the conversation, refocusing priorities or facilitating access to resources. Patient activisms claim "the right to participate in the social processes through which science and technology evolve" (Blume, 1997, p. 51). HIV-positive patients challenged policy and research agendas in the 1980s to gain access to treatments (Epstein, 1995), as did some of the earlier advocates for breast cancer research (Klawiter, 2002, 2004; Kolker, 2004). Cochlear implants for deaf children, for which there have been "rhetorics and counter-rhetorics" (Blume, 1997, 1999), generated biosocial *resistance* to new health technologies, but many biomedical treatments have motivated movements that embrace new technologies as empowering. The advocacy against Gardasil's policies drew upon existing mechanisms of authority, failing to question Perry's presumed biomedical categories. Rather than advocates *for* health improvements, these groups defined themselves as opponents.

The responses to RP 65 differ from other late 20th-century patient-oriented activism, organized around health-specific collective identities. Distinct from influential HIV or breast cancer patient advocates, for whom health conditions have served as political and social identities, the RP 65 opponents *rejected* the new health technology. Suspicion of Gardasil policy focused less on proposed health benefits, reducing HPV morbidity and potential cancer through vaccination, than on Perry's political maneuvers and government power. Although groups like PROVE doubted Gardasil's population-level health benefits, no objections to RP 65 offered alternatives to defend claims that the vaccine had limited urgency. For example, improved access to cervical cancer screening or enhanced resources for women's health could serve as moderately persuasive substitutes to vaccination. RP 65 opponents barely addressed health outcomes, preoccupied with questions of power and authority.

Merck's influence on legislation

Gardasil policy opponents included parents who accepted other school entry vaccines. Critics of vaccines often present "gradations of acceptance" (Streefland et al., 1999) and may not reject all vaccines categorically. Few parents contended explicitly with Gardasil's medical or scientific data[7] but focused on whether states *could require* vaccines and argued parental preferences should trump policy. Anthropological and sociological research demonstrate that parents' anxieties about vaccines include fearing their children are guinea pigs for big pharma or distrusting pharmaceutical financial motivations (Gottlieb, 2015; Leach & Fairhead, 2007). Parental skepticism of business interests were not irrational reactions to the sudden legislative push but may be understood as astute responses to legitimate corporate machinations.[8]

Merck strategically avoided sexual health politics by defining Gardasil as a cancer vaccine. Merck met with conservative family groups in 2005 to promote Gardasil's cancer protection as a preemptive move before FDA review. These groups expressed concern that the vaccine would be made 'mandatory' (Steenhuysen, 2006). The cancer emphasis initially muted any resistance from conservative family organizations:

> "This is an awesome vaccine," [said] Linda Klepacki, analyst for sexual health at Focus on the Family. . . . "It could prevent millions of deaths around the world. We support this vaccine. We see it as an extremely important medical breakthrough." What they are against, she explained, is making vaccination mandatory rather than leaving it up to parents to decide. (Gibbs, 2006)

Yet, after cultivating conservative groups' support, Merck made the strange decision to lobby state legislatures (Gardner, 2007; Pollack & Saul, 2007) and the group Women in Government (WIG), a "non-profit, bi-partisan[9] organization of women federal and state legislators" (Women in Government 2008). In 2004, WIG developed its "Challenge to Eliminate Cervical Cancer," which, according to their website, expanded their March 2003 summit, "HPV and Cervical Cancer Task Force Meeting" (Women in Government 2008). The timing of WIG's interest in cervical cancer, prior to Gardasil's FDA review, may suggest they championed preventive women's health legislation. But a more likely explanation is that Merck and GlaxoSmithKline provided WIG financial/educational support for their 2003–2004 cervical cancer symposia, which coincided with the development of Gardasil and Cervarix. Indeed, as one pharmaceutical marketing magazine observed, "as early as 2003, the firm [Merck] was laying the groundwork with a global education campaign aimed at helping patients and healthcare professionals draw the link between HPV and cervical cancer" (Arnold, 2008, p. 46). WIG allows corporations to have direct access to its politician members. Its president, Susan Crosby, acknowledged willingness to accept funds from Merck, emphasizing that their multiple corporate sponsors provided unbiased information to legislators, "I don't see it as a conflict of interest because they're not funding a particular legislator or a particular mission . . . I would say that if you know our women legislators . . . you know that no one particular person or industry is going to tell them or dictate to them what they're going to do" (Siers-Poisson, 2008). Merck's lobbying, though notable, is part of the established political–private sector collaboration. In 2001, for example, Merck met with the FDA to discuss its cervical cancer vaccine development, which would prioritize precancerous stages as the target end point for a vaccine (FDA, 2006). Growing public awareness that corporations influence all levels of political and regulatory bodies suggests that there are few authoritative institutions without corporate ties (Lenzer, 2015). This ubiquity does not mean corporate influence transparency is not necessary; rather, it suggests it is critical.

After RP 65: Gardasil today

Texas legislators introduced their policy protest to RP 65, H.B. 1098, to the state House of Representatives two days after Perry's executive order (KXAN .com, 2007) and introduced another similar bill, H.B. 1115 (2007), on February 12. On February 20, 2007, in Austin, Texas, a public hearing considered H.B. 1098 to rescind RP 65. H.B. 1098 declared school attendance did not require the HPV vaccine. The proponents of H.B. 1098 defined the bill in contrast to Perry's use of executive authority and in terms of an imagined threat of sexual promiscuity.

> The bill [1098] would maintain the ability of parents to control the upbringing of their children. Executive order RP-65 [sic] would undermine the ability of parents to control their children's health care. The opt-out program in RP-65 [sic] is complicated and unclear. The mandatory vaccination also could in some cases encourage young women to engage in early sexual activity by giving them the false impression that immunity from the HPV virus makes all sexual activity safer and more acceptable (House Research Organization, 2007, p. 3).

On February 21, less than three weeks after Perry's order and a day after the introduction of H.B. 1098, Merck announced its decision to cease nationwide lobbying in response to parents (Pollack & Saul, 2007). Merck formally stated lobbying "could undermine adoption of the vaccine" (Pollack & Saul, 2007), but the announcement during the Texas debates suggests they informed Merck's decision. Although lobbying for pharmaceutical interests is a common practice in the U.S., other pharmaceutical products do not lead to state or federal requirements. Antidepressants or antibiotics do not have policies requiring people of a certain age or sex receive treatment, nor do they trigger immigrant citizenship standards. The cascading effects of Merck's and Perry's maneuvers call attention to the power of vaccines in policy and public health interventions.

During the 2012 presidential primary season, Rick Perry's executive order became a topic for debate among his fellow Republican contenders. Another candidate, Michele Bachmann, argued the HPV vaccine was unsafe, although her claims had no scientific evidence (Huisenga, 2011). During Perry's first presidential campaign, he acknowledged, for the first time, that his executive order was a mistake, addressing citizen involvement in health-care policy: "The fact of the matter is that I didn't do my research well enough to understand that we needed to have a substantial conversation with our citizenry" (Eggen, 2011). Perry understood his contentious order as a problem of public discourse and the limits of executive authority, not as a problem of vaccine efficacy, nor about health concerns at all.

No one has definitively proven that Gardasil's early policies, with RP 65 the most contentious, have affected uptake of HPV vaccines, but data show its coverage lags well behind other adolescent and childhood vaccination rates (CDC, 2014; Elam-Evans et al., 2014). Most recent CDC data, collected seven years after FDA approval, reveal fewer than 50% of boys have received all three shots of HPV vaccine, and only 70% of girls have completed their series (Elam-Evans et al., 2014). These numbers contrast starkly to other standard vaccines, including the controversial measles-mumps-rubella vaccine, which more than 90% of adolescents have received (Elam-Evans et al., 2014). Rather than motivating parents to choose Gardasil for their daughters (and eventually their sons), the state legislatures' failed policies heightened parental distrust. Pharmaceutical companies' marketing and strategic positionings are not unique to vaccines, but also few vaccines have the marketing push of Gardasil; private sector interests combined with widespread public policy initiatives made parents wary.

Gardasil arrived at a moment when vaccine distrust became part of a broader public discourse, not just voiced by skeptical outliers. As more parents opt out of some or all vaccines, they call attention to how "the new political economy of vitality ... [is] coupled with local intensifications and regulated by supra-national institutions" (Rabinow & Rose, 2006, p. 215). Jenny McCarthy, a vocal public opponent of the current vaccine schedule, and her 2007 appearance on Oprah's television show transformed vaccine resistance into a mainstream topic (Gottlieb, 2015). In 2008 and 2015, U.S. measles outbreaks (CDC, 2008, 2015) led to public health concerns about increasing numbers of U.S. parents opting out of some or all vaccines. Rising rates of pertussis in California, also known as whooping cough, have been attributed to declining vaccination (Atwell et al., 2013), although there may be other reasons for its resurgence (Blume & Zanders, 2006). Legislating Gardasil occurred concurrently with parents deliberately deploying legal strategies to resist state vaccine policies.

At the same time, as the Texas case reveals, the HPV vaccines are different from other vaccines. Gardasil's association with an STI makes it a unique vaccine. This may explain the parents' lawsuits, the swift, successful opposition to Perry's order, and the federal Gingrey bill, as well as Merck's relative market failure in spite of carefully crafted cancer claims.[10] Merck's financially motivated policy push and Perry's other restrictive women's health policies in Texas suggest that women's best interests were never the priority of Gardasil distribution. Over the last decade, the Texas government has restricted funds to organizations like Planned Parenthood (Culp-Ressler, 2015; Tan, 2011), resulting in defunded breast and cervical cancer screening programs, central to Planned Parenthood's mission to improve women's health. The policies also exclude Texas from receiving federal funds to support preventive screenings. Perry's pro-life claim to preserve women's health did not extend to already sexually active women at more imminent risk for life-threatening cancers.

As vaccines' targets extend beyond airborne contagions, the self-evident benefits of vaccine technologies become less persuasive for those who raise concerns (Leach & Fairhead, 2007). Widespread (and continued) vaccination successfully controls contagious infections, but the newer vaccines, such as for varicella (chickenpox), are perceived as less critical than older vaccines for life-threatening diseases. As vaccination policies become more restrictive, with state legislations eliminating non-medical exemptions (Krieger & Calefati, 2015; McGreevy, 2015), vaccine anxieties manifest through resistances and refusals. The 2007 response in Texas presaged ongoing U.S. vaccine policy debates. Yet, although parents with children who cannot receive vaccines due to age or immune-compromised conditions might advocate for broad vaccination requirements, there is no corollary advocacy for Gardasil. It has been marketed as an individual intervention, even as it, too, is for a communicable virus.

Gardasil raises the important question of how might it have been otherwise? This chapter has only briefly explored the reasons *to require* the vaccine because it is unclear whether this *ought to* be a required U.S. vaccine. Its utility to prevent cervical cancer mortality in the U.S. is limited, given current rates of cervical cancer screening. Its protection against other types of sexually transmitted cancers, which lack standard screening practices, has great potential, but this would require a significant shift in male sexual health management. Gardasil can reduce HPV-related morbidity, which will save women from unnecessary suffering and stigma. But not once in the Texas or national discourse about the vaccine's value to women have public officials emphasized these benefits. Prior to Gardasil's FDA approval, Merck subsidized a number of HPV-awareness education projects (Arnold, 2008), none of which still exist years after Gardasil's launch (Gottlieb, 2013, forthcoming). Gardasil remains a vaccine with little public demand.

Gardasil, in its earlier quadrivalent and current nonavalent incarnations, occupies a tenuous place in health interventions. It is a vaccine and an STI preventive, offering cancer-based prevention for those inoculated young enough to avoid exposure to cancerous HPV. Its multiplicity, as an STI intervention *and* as a vaccine, taps into fraught discourses about regulating specific bodies, anticipations of nascent sexual individuals, and parents' perceived loss of control over their children as they reach adulthood. Legislative maneuvers, hastened and encouraged by Merck, only diminished parents' acceptance of a population-wide Gardasil vaccine requirement. Perry, along with Merck, laid bare corporate complicity in capitalizing on population health interventions. Gardasil offers a distinct example of biomedical resistances: parental resistance within biopower's framework, *not* as a rejection of institutional authority. The case of Gardasil in its first years after FDA approval forces us to ask, When rejecting biomedical legislation with counter-legislation, what do we call this form of refusal? Are there certain contexts in which biopower's reach may make non-institutional refusals nearly impossible?

Editor commentary

In this provocative piece exploring parental resistance to the Gardasil vaccine in the U.S. state of Texas, Samantha Gottlieb argues:

1. Parental concern over this vaccine was unique in that it was less about vaccine content than other counter-vaccine arguments in the past.
2. Resistance increases when policies become more restrictive.
3. Identifying particular sectors of the population (young women, non-citizens) to receive a communally beneficial health intervention raises social concerns that counter scientific argument.
4. Resistances in this case be considered a reaction to participation in biopower's multiplicity.

In addition, this piece

- explains and draws upon the theoretical perspectives of *biopower* (the use of government institutions to control human vitality, morbidity, and mortality) and *biosociality* (the generation of a social identity based on biological conditions);
- highlights that technologies are not neutral entities but imbued with social, political, historic, and economic meanings;
- notes that public responses to new technologies are unpredictable and that new biomedical technologies can be seen as concurrently restrictive and empowering;
- argues that involvement of citizenry in the development and establishment of public health policy is imperative; and
- asserts that public demand for health technologies is an important driver of innovation and policy.

Notes

1 Medicalization describes the increasing range of human activities that health and medical management target (Lock, 2001; Moynihan, Heath, & Henry, 2002; Zola, 1972).

2 Teixeira and Löwy (2011) contest whether the Pap smear must necessarily be the reason that cervical cancer mortality has dropped, an important critique of deterministic assumptions about healthcare interventions, but this will not be explored here.

3 I question Gardasil's revolutionary promise elsewhere (Gottlieb, 2013, forthcoming).

4 Insufficient data on males reflect long-standing gendered practices in reproductive and sexual health medicine; sexual health has traditionally focused on women for surveillance and regulation. No marketed test for HPV in men exists, and men do not have institutionalized sexual health maintenance like women. Therefore, data on and awareness of HPV in men remain lacking. Due to space limitations, these will not be explored here.

5 The court's structure is partly to protect pharmaceutical companies from the risk of high-cost litigation, as well as to cap injury claims. Companies have claimed they would otherwise be disincentivized to produce vaccines.

6 Now known as Immigration Customs Enforcement (ICE).

7 In other U.S. parental vaccine resistances, vaccine ingredients and safety are often the focus.
8 Recent research revealed the CDC receives considerable donations from pharmaceutical corporations. This casts its public reputation as "an independent watchdog over the public health" in doubt (Lenzer, 2015, p. 1).
9 Note this is not *non*partisan.
10 Media coverage of Gardasil before market launch anticipated a blockbuster product (Arnold 2008), which has yet to materialize.

References

Adams, P. (2012). Reaching teenagers with three-times jab is a first for most countries. *Bulletin of the World Health Organization*, *90*(12), 874–875.

Adams, V., Murphy, M., & Clarke, A. E. (2009). Anticipation: Technoscience, life, affect, temporality. *Subjectivity*, *28*(1), 246–265.

Allen, A. (2007). *Vaccine: The Controversial Story of Medicine's Greatest Lifesaver*. New York: W.W. Norton & Company.

Anonymous. (2007). Statement of Gov. Rick Perry on HPV Vaccine Executive Order. *La Prensa*, p. 18.

Arnold, M. (2008). MM&M All-Stars Company of the Year: Merck. *Medical Marketing and Media, 1 January 2008*.

Atwell, J., Van Otterloo, J., Zipprich, J., Winter, K., Harriman, K., Salmon, D., . . . Omer, S. (2013). Nonmedical vaccine exemptions and pertussis in California, 2010. *Pediatrics*, *132*(4), 624–630.

Baer, H., Allen, S., & Braun, L. (2000). Knowledge of human papillomavirus infection among young adult men and women: Implications for health education and research. *Journal of Community Health*, *25*(1), 67–78.

Blinder, A. (2015). Mississippi, a Vaccination Leader, Stands by Its Strict Rules. *New York Times*, 4 February 2015.

Blume, S. (1997). The rhetoric and counter-rhetoric of a "bionic" technology. *Science, Technology & Human Values*, *22*(1), 31–56.

Blume, S. (1999). Histories of cochlear implantation. *Social Science & Medicine*, *49*(9), 1257–1268.

Blume, S., & Zanders, M. (2006). Vaccine independence, local competences and globalisation: Lessons from the history of pertussis vaccines. *Social Science & Medicine*, *63*(7), 1825–1835.

Blumenthal, B. (2007). Texas Is First to Require Cancer Shots for Schoolgirls. *New York Times*, 3 February 2007.

Browner, C. H., & Press, N. (1996). The production of authoritative knowledge in American prenatal care. *Medical Anthropology Quarterly*, *10*(2), 141–156.

CDC. (2008). Outbreak of measles – San Diego, California, January–February 2008. *Morbidity and Mortality Weekly Report*, *57*(8), 203–206.

CDC. (2014). Human papillomavirus vaccination coverage among adolescents, 2007–2013, and postlicensure vaccine safety monitoring, 2006–2014 – United States. *Morbidity and Mortality Weekly Report*, *63*(29), 620–624.

CDC. (2015). Measles: Cases and Outbreaks. Retrieved from http://www.cdc.gov/measles/cases-outbreaks.html

Clarke, A., Shim, J. K., Mamo, L., & Fosket, J. R. (2003). Biomedicalization: Technoscientific transformations of health, illness, and US biomedicine. *American Sociological Review*, *68*(2), 161–194.

Coe, E. (2007). Merck Vaccine Sparks Lawsuit. Law360.com.

Colgrove, J. (2006). *State of Immunity: The Politics of Vaccination in Twentieth-Century America*. New York: University of California Press.

Culp-Ressler, T. (2015). Texas May Slash Cancer Screenings for Low-Income Women. Retrieved from www.thinkprogress.org/health/2015/01/29/3617158/texas-budget-cancer-planned-parenthood/

D'Urso, J., Thompson-Robinson, M., & Chandler, S. (2007). HPV knowledge and behaviors of black college students at a historically black university. *Journal of American College Health*, *56*(2), 159–163.

Dimond, R., Bartlett, A., & Lewis, J. (2015). What binds biosociality? The collective effervescence of the parent-led conference. *Social Science & Medicine*, *126*, 1–8.

Donzelot, J. (1979). *The Policing of Families*. New York: Pantheon.

Eggen, D. (2011, 13 September). Rick Perry Reverses Himself, Calls HPV Vaccine Mandate a 'Mistake'. *Washington Post*.

Elam-Evans, L., Yankey, D., Jeyarajah, J., Singleton, J., Curtis, C., MacNeil, J., & Hariri, S. (2014). National, regional, state, and selected local area vaccination coverage among adolescents aged 13–17 years – United States, 2013. *Morbidity and Mortality Weekly Report*, *63*(29), 625–633.

Epstein, S. (1995). The construction of lay expertise: AIDS activism and the forging of credibility in the reform of clinical trials. *Science, Technology & Human Values*, *20*(4), 408–437.

FDA. (2006). Center for Biologics Evaluation and Research, Vaccines and Related Biological Products Advisory Meeting (Vol. 18 May 2006). Washington, DC: Food and Drug Administration.

FDA. (2009). Press Release, FDA Approves New Indication for Gardasil to Prevent Genital Warts in Men and Boys (Vol. 16 October 2009). Washington, DC: Food and Drug Administration.

FDA. (2010). Press Release, FDA: Gardasil Approved to Prevent Anal Cancer (Vol. 22 December 2010). Washington, DC: Food and Drug Administration.

Foucault, M., & Ewald, F. (2003). *Society Must Be Defended: Lectures at the Collège de France, 1975–1976*. New York: Macmillan.

Friedman, A., & Shepeard, H. (2007). Exploring the knowledge, attitudes, beliefs, and communication preferences of the general public regarding HPV findings from CDC focus group research and implications for practice. *Health Education & Behavior*, *34*(3), 471–485.

Gardner, A. (2007). Drugmaker Assists in Pushing for Mandate for HPV Vaccination. http://www.washingtonpost.com/wp-dyn/content/article/2007/02/10/AR2007021001279.html.

Gibbs, N. (2006). Defusing the War over the "Promiscuity" Vaccine. *Time*, June 21, 2006.

Gottlieb, S. D. (2013). The patient-consumer-advocate nexus: The marketing and dissemination of Gardasil, the human papillomavirus vaccine in the United States. *Medical Anthropology Quarterly*, *27*(3), 330–347.

Gottlieb, S. D. (2015). Vaccine resistances reconsidered: Vaccine skeptics and the Jenny McCarthy effect. *BioSocieties*. doi:10.1057/biosoc.2015.30

Gottlieb, S. D. (forthcoming). *Not Quite a Cancer Vaccine: The Marketing of Merck's HPV Vaccine*. Retrieved from http://www.academia.edu/23060653/_forthcoming_Not_Quite_a_Cancer_Vaccine_The_Marketing_of_the_HPV_Vaccine.

Grissom, B. (2007, 24 February). 3 Families Sue Perry Over HPV Mandate. *El Paso Times*.

Grosz, E. (1994). *Volatile Bodies: Toward a Corporeal Feminism*. Bloomington: Indiana University Press.

Haddix, A. (2009). Criteria for vaccination requirements for U.S. immigration purposes. *Federal Register*, *74*, 218.

Hands Off Our Kids Coalition. (2007). Letter to Texas Governor, Re: HPV Vaccine Mandate. Retrieved from www.vaccineinfo.net/immunization/vaccine/hpv/index.shtml

Harris, G. (2006a, 30 June). Panel Unanimously Recommends Cervical Cancer Vaccine for Girls 11 and Up. *New York Times.*

Harris, G. (2006b, 8 June). U.S. Approves Cervical Cancer Vaccine. *New York Times.*

Harris, G. (2008, 8 March). Deal in an Autism Case Fuels Debate on Vaccine. *New York Times.*

H.B. 215. (2007). *An Act Relating to Immunization Against Human Papilloma Virus.*

H.B. 1098. (2007). *Act Relating to Immunization Against Human Papillomavirus.*

H.R. 1153. (2007). *Parental Right to Decide Protection Act.*

Hobson-West, P. (2003). Understanding vaccination resistance: Moving beyond risk. *Health, Risk & Society, 5*(3), 273–283.

Hodge, J. (2002). School Vaccination Requirements: Legal and Social Perspectives. *NCSL State Legislative Report, August 2002.* Washington, DC: National Conference of State Legislatures.

House Research Organization. (2007). Bill Analysis, Prohibiting Mandatory Immunization Against Human Papilloma Virus. Retrieved from www.hro.house.state.tx.us/pdf/ba80r/hb1098.pdf

Huisenga, S. (2011). PAC backing Bachmann continues HPV vaccine claims. *National Journal, 21* September 2011.

Jasanoff, S. (2004). Science and citizenship: A new synergy. *Science and Public Policy, 31*(2), 90–94.

Jemal, A., Bray, F., Center, M., Ferlay, J., Ward, E., & Forman, D. (2011). Global cancer statistics. *CA: A Cancer Journal for Clinicians, 61*(2), 69–90.

Johnson, L. (2007, 2 February). Cancer Vaccine Faces Cost Hurdles. *AP News.*

Kapsalis, T. (1997). *Public Privates: Performing Gynecology from Both Ends of the Speculum.* Durham: Duke University Press.

Klawiter, M. (2002). Risk, prevention and the breast cancer continuum: The NCI, the FDA, health activism and the pharmaceutical industry. *History and Technology, 18*(4), 309–353.

Klawiter, M. (2004). Breast cancer in two regimes: The impact of social movements on illness experience. *Sociology of Health & Illness, 26*(6), 845–874.

Klug, S., Hukelmann, M., & Blettner, M. (2008). Knowledge about infection with human papillomavirus: A systematic review. *Preventive Medicine, 46*(2), 87–98.

Kolker, E. (2004). Framing as a cultural resource in health social movements: Funding activism and the breast cancer movement in the US 1990–1993. *Sociology of Health & Illness, 26*(6), 820–844.

Krieger, L. M., & Calefati, J. (2015, 5 February). Measles outbreak: Vaccination Exemption Would End under Proposed California Law. *San Jose Mercury News.* Retrieved from http://www.mercurynews.com/health/ci_27458564/measles-california-outbreak-vaccination-exemption-religious-belief

KXAN.com. (2007). Public Hearing on HPV Vaccine Went until Midnight. kxan.com, Retrieved 21 February 2007.

Leach, M., & Fairhead, J. (2007). *Vaccine Anxieties: Global Science, Child Health, and Society.* New York: Routledge.

Lehoux, P., & Blume, S. (2000). Technology assessment and the sociopolitics of health technologies. *Journal of Health Politics Policy and Law, 25*(6), 1083–1120.

Lenzer, J. (2015). Centers for Disease Control and Prevention: Protecting the private good? *British Medical Journal, 350,* h2362.

Lock, M. (2001). The tempering of medical anthropology: Troubling natural categories. *Medical Anthropology Quarterly, 15*(4), 478–492.

Longoria, T. (2008, 27 September). Human Papillomavirus Vaccination Requirement for Immigrants Raises Concerns. *Dallas Morning News*.

Mamo, L., & Epstein, S. (2014). The pharmaceuticalization of sexual risk: Vaccine development and the new politics of cancer prevention. *Social Science & Medicine, 101*, 155–165.

Martin, E. (2001). *The Woman in the Body: A Cultural Analysis of Reproduction*. Boston: Beacon Press.

McGreevy, P. (2015, 4 February). Bill Would Abolish Vaccination Exemption for Parents' Personal Beliefs. *Los Angeles Times*.

Moynihan, R., Heath, I., & Henry, D. (2002). Selling sickness: The pharmaceutical industry and disease mongering. Commentary: Medicalisation of risk factors. *British Medical Journal, 324*(7342), 886–891.

Muñoz, N., Castellsagué, X., de González, A., & Gissmann, L. (2006). HPV in the etiology of human cancer. *Vaccine, 24*, S1–S10.

National Conference of State Legislatures. (2007). HPV Vaccine Policies. Retrieved from www.ncsl.org/research/health/hpv-vaccine-state-legislation-and-statutes.aspx#2006

Offit, P. (2008, 31 March). Inoculated against Facts. *New York Times*.

Oudshoorn, N. (2003). *The Male Pill: A Biography of a Technology in the Making*. Durham: Duke University Press.

Parthasarathy, S. (2005). Architectures of genetic medicine comparing genetic testing for breast cancer in the USA and the UK. *Social Studies of Science, 35*(1), 5–40.

Perry, R. (2007). Executive Order RP 65, 2 February, 2007.

Pollack, A., & Saul, S. (2007, 21 February). Merck to Halt Lobbying for Vaccine for Girls. *New York Times*.

Pollitt, K. (2005, 30 May). Virginity or Death! *The Nation*.

Rabinow, P. (1984). *The Foucault Reader: An Introduction to Foucault's Thought, with Major New Unpublished Material*. London: Penguin.

Rabinow, P., & Rose, N. (2006). Biopower today. *BioSocieties, 1*(2), 195–217.

Rapp, R. (2001). Gender, body, biomedicine: How some feminist concerns dragged reproduction to the center of social theory. *Medical Anthropology Quarterly, 15*(4), 466–477.

S.B. 110. (2007). *An Act Relating to Immunization against Human Papilloma Virus*.

S.B. 438. (2007). *An Act Relating to Prohibiting Immunization against Human Papilloma Virus As a Condition for Admission to Public School*.

Schwartz, J. L., Caplan, A. L., Faden, R. R., & Sugarman, J. (2007). Lessons from the failure of human papillomavirus vaccine state requirements. *Clinical Pharmacology & Therapeutics, 82*(6), 760–763.

Siers-Poisson, J. (2008). Women in Government, Merck's Trojan Horse: Series on the Politics and PR of Cervical Cancer. *Center for Media and Democracy*. Retrieved from www.prwatch.org/node/6232/

Singh, G. (2012). Rural–urban trends and patterns in cervical cancer mortality, incidence, stage, and survival in the United States, 1950–2008. *Journal of Community Health, 37*(1), 217–223.

Steenhuysen, J. (2006, 22 June). Merck Cancer Vaccine Faces Christian Right Scrutiny. *Reuters*.

Streefland, P., Chowdhury, A., & Ramos-Jimenez, P. (1999). Patterns of vaccination acceptance. *Social Science & Medicine, 49*(12), 1705–1716.

Tan, T. (2011). Day 15: Texas Family Planning Funding Slashed. *Texas Tribune*. Retrieved from www.texastribune.org/2011/08/15/day-15/

Teixiera, L. A., & Löwy, I. (2011). Imperfect tools for a difficult job: Colposcopy, "colpocytology" and screening for cervical cancer in Brazil. *Social Studies of Science, 41*, 585–608.

Tell Someone. (2006). Merck & Co., Inc. Television advertisement.

Thompson, M. (2010). Who's guarding what? A poststructural feminist analysis of Gardasil discourses. *Health Communication*, *25*(2), 119–130.

VaccineInfo.net. (2007). Alert – Oppose Forced HPV Vaccine on Girls in Texas. Retrieved from www.vaccineinfo.net/immunization/vaccine/hpv/index.shtml

Van Kammen, J. (1999). Representing users' bodies: The gendered development of anti-fertility vaccines. *Science, Technology & Human Values*, *24*(3), 307–337.

Wynn, L., & Trussell, J. (2006). The social life of emergency contraception in the United States: Disciplining pharmaceutical use, disciplining sexuality, and constructing zygotic bodies. *Medical Anthropology Quarterly*, *20*(3), 297–320.

Zola, I. (1972). Medicine as an institution of social control. *The Sociological Review*, *20*(4), 487–504.

4

RESISTANCE OR PARASITISM?

Waste Scavengers and Dengue Mosquito Control in Nicaragua

Alex M. Nading

Ciudad Sandino, Nicaragua, a community of over 100,000 residents just north of Managua, is home to plenty of mosquitoes, and it contains plenty of places for them to hide and breed. Ciudad Sandino is divided into 14 neighborhoods, known as *zonas*. The zonas are comprised of uniform 10 × 30 m house lots, each directly abutting the next. *Aedes aegypti* mosquitoes, which transmit the dengue virus among humans, prefer to breed in such close-knit spaces. Female *Ae. aegypti* tend to lay their eggs in water basins, sinks, gutters, and sometimes in accumulated household waste. The adult female of the species is capable of carrying the dengue virus, which has become a growing public health threat across urban Latin America. Indeed, dengue is so common in urban Nicaragua that most human adults – whether or not they know it – have likely been exposed to the virus by the time they reach 20 years of age (Standish, et al. 2010). The dengue virus infects over 250 million people per year, from Singapore to South Florida. It is the most prevalent mosquito-borne disease in the world.

This chapter draws on fieldwork I conducted in Ciudad Sandino between 2006 and 2011 to discuss the relationship of household waste to global dengue prevention strategies (Nading, 2014). In Ciudad Sandino, where formal unemployment ranges from 50% to 75%, scavenging and selling recyclable materials is a common livelihood strategy (Hartmann, 2012). The garbage trade is a frequent target of Nicaragua's national dengue control policy. In 2008, an ongoing political struggle over waste management in Ciudad Sandino became entangled with an ongoing dengue fever epidemic. By tracing this entanglement, I argue that the relationship between local populations and global health initiatives might best be seen not as one of binary domination and resistance but of multidirectional "parasitism" (Serres, 2007 [1982]). In Ciudad Sandino's urban waste controversy, global dengue prevention policy was certainly at issue, but it was almost never *directly* addressed by the actors involved.

Source reduction

I am trudging slowly behind a garbage truck as it winds through Zona 10. At first, the process of collection seems familiar and tedious. *Recolectores* (they are all men) pick up bags of refuse in each house, transfer their contents to a truck or trailer bed, and walk off to the next house. Things get more interesting when the truck bed fills up. That is when we load up and drive to the municipal dump.

Ciudad Sandino's dump is a disused farm field. There are two ways in and out. One is by municipal vehicle – usually a white Toyota dump truck. Garbage truck drivers prefer to go in and out rapidly. In the dry season, this means that the *recolectores* who ride atop the mounds of refuse in the exposed bed become shrouded in a fine red dust. In the rainy season, the trucks splash through mud puddles, and chances are high that the vehicles will become stuck in the furrows of the dump, which sits adjacent to an outlying zona called Nueva Vida.

Before unloading the garbage, most crews make a quick stop on the entrance road that divides the field from Nueva Vida. There, the *recolectores* in the truck bed jump out and jog into a nearby house, a structure made of wood and sheet metal surrounded by a flimsy fence of immature tree trunks and a few strands of rusty barbed wire. The *recolectores* haul massive plastic grain sacks filled with their day's catch of *chatarra. Chatarra,* literally "junk," is the omnibus term in Nicaragua for recyclable materials, from plastic bottles to cans, copper wiring, scrap iron, and paper. A woman in the house will weigh and buy these items. While awaiting payment from the buyer (or *chatarrero*), the *recolectores* might cross paths with garbage scavengers like Doña Flor, a fiftyish woman who works in the dump picking out the recyclables that the crews leave behind.

On this day, I decide to say good-bye to the truck and crew and accompany Doña Flor, the garbage scavenger, to her house. She leads me on the other route out of the dump and into Nueva Vida. She walks slowly, a spiked metal prod for sifting through rubbish piles balanced on her shoulder. For me, her pace through the barrio, shaded from the sun that scorches the treeless dump, is as refreshing in its ease as the rides on the garbage trucks were in their briskness. She shares her house with two sons and a few grandchildren. This house, too, has a flimsy barbed wire fence enclosing piles of recyclables. The piles grow and shrink inversely with the market prices of the materials they contain.

Over the weeks and months, recyclables move in and out of her house and in and out of Ciudad Sandino in a waste stream that flows from scavengers to small buyers, on to large brokers in Managua, and ultimately to faraway ports on other continents. The stream bears money, people, and product brand identities. Insects also ride along. *Ae. aegypti* mosquitoes sometimes lay eggs in the things Doña Flor and others collect.

Ae. aegypti is more difficult to control than its malaria-spreading distant cousins in genus *Anopheles* because it occupies the intimate, private spaces people call home. Given its adaptability to households and their surroundings, controlling *Ae. Aegypti* – and thus controlling dengue fever – requires, first, that communities have effective water and waste management. Second, someone must inform individuals about the mosquito and its breeding habits and convince them that they should be on the lookout for potential breeding sites. In the absence of an effective dengue vaccine, these two priorities – waste/water management and mosquito control – have made a house-to-house mosquito "source reduction" strategy the only globally accepted strategy for preventing dengue. The goal of this strategy is to make the urban environment unwelcoming to the mosquito by encouraging people, through a combination of insecticide application, public education, and law enforcement, to rid their homes of potential breeding sites, or "sources," including waste.

This approach dates back to the earliest days of mosquito control, and it hinges on a feedback between perceptions of collective risk and personal responsibility (Beck, 1992; Carter, 2012; Peterson & Lupton, 1996). Managing this feedback has long been a key part of maintaining public health across Latin America. As Charles Briggs and Clara Mantini-Briggs suggest, ideas about who is capable of contemplating and acting on health risk and who, by dint of racial, ethnic, or gendered discrimination, is doomed to be victimized or demonized, constitute a domain of "sanitary citizenship" (2003, pp. 319–320). In the case of dengue, the making of sanitary citizens means fostering a recognition that things, people, and mosquitoes are entangled, and determining differing levels of responsibility for managing that entanglement (Nading, 2012).

During my fieldwork, I witnessed dozens of campaigns led by the Nicaraguan Ministry of Health (Ministerio de Salud, henceforth, MINSA) in which doctors, garbage collectors, and community health workers (*brigadistas*) exhorted homeowners to discard the plastic, rubber, and scrap metal piled in their homes. Brigadistas walked alongside the garbage trucks, reminding residents that mosquitoes like to breed in the pools of rainwater that form in those piles, and that there was neither a cure nor an effective vaccine for dengue. They spoke vividly about the consequences of inaction: the spread of a virus that causes hemorrhagic fevers, physical impairment, and even death. But the campaigns failed to create a consensus among residents about how to stop dengue from spreading. Instead, they aggravated social divisions among health workers, city garbage collectors, and garbage scavengers. These divisions arose not over how to define the disease (no one disputed that dengue was a problem) but over how to foster community participation, how to manage space, and how to balance resources and hazards. In short, they were about the limits to sanitary citizenship.

In Ciudad Sandino, as in other places, waste has long been a focus of source reduction efforts, whether in one-off cleanup campaigns or in more routine house-to-house mosquito control efforts. While some have posited links between inadequate solid waste control and dengue, those links tend to be oversimplified. Studies tend to characterize the wastes that can become mosquito-breeding sites as problems typical of "consumer societies" (Ashencaenen-Crabtree, Wong, & Mas'ud, 2001; Gubler, 1989). Discourses about the "choice" to scavenge or otherwise harbor garbage that might play host to mosquitoes spin an "apolitical" narrative of dengue ecology (Robbins, 2012). What is missing is an investigation of how global economic pressures and social relationships entangle the social lives of mosquitoes and people with those of non-living materials, making the ideal of sanitary citizenship impossible to achieve.

Disturbances to garbage economies, disease ecologies

The year 2008 saw two turning points in the relationships between Ciudad Sandino's garbage scavengers, its mosquitoes, and the Nicaraguan state. The first turning point came in March, when scavengers organized blockades of the dumps in Ciudad Sandino and nearby Managua. Until 2006, the scavengers had a nearly uncontested claim to garbage of value, but persistent poverty and a spike in global demand for recyclables changed both the geography and the demography of scavenging. From late 2005 to mid-2008, worldwide prices for recyclable materials soared. City garbage collectors, whose work gave them easy access to the waste stream, took special advantage of the boom, picking up large amounts of plastic, metal, and aluminum on their daily routes. This on-route recycling sparked the scavengers' protests. For several days, they lobbed rocks at city vehicles that dared to enter the dumps. They demanded that city leaders order garbage collectors to stop selecting and selling recyclables during their work routes (Hartmann, 2012).

Both scavengers and garbage collectors recognized not only that without their labor, recyclables could not realize their market value, but also that without their efforts, the city could not come close to being clean. Although both groups tried to secure exclusive access to garbage of value, neither found a satisfying way to convince the city government that it deserved rights to collect. Both groups were trying to secure their positions as what scholars of Latin American politics call "clients" to powerful "patrons" in the city government. Elaborated in the post-independence period, the concept of patron–clientelism helps explain how wealth and power become distributed systematically across spaces that government institutions cannot reach. In the ideal-typical version, "patrons" use wealth and generosity to mobilize the labor of poorer clients, who reciprocate with political loyalty. Importantly, individuals may play the role of both patron and client simultaneously. A small-time patron may in turn be the client of an even more powerful person. At each level, people sacrifice their individual rights as citizens for material goods. A system based on patron–clientelism – as Ciudad Sandino's garbage economy largely was – is somewhat at odds with ideas of sanitary citizenship, as well as with a free and open market. The scavengers saw city leaders' tacit approval of the garbage collectors' actions as a violation of an implied moral contract. They, not the collectors, deserved to pick up the city's valuable wastes.

But the situation was not that simple. Though the garbage collectors appeared to hold familiar, modern public works jobs, they depended on strong relationships with political bosses for their job security. Civic leaders, likewise, needed someone to keep the city minimally clean. Their patronage was not simple generosity. They, too, depended on formal and informal garbage collectors to validate their own political legitimacy.

If the dump conflict marked the first turning point in the relationships between garbage scavengers, mosquitoes, and the state, then the Plan Chatarra, a nationwide campaign devised by MINSA in 2008 to ban scavenging and garbage trading from city centers and relegate it to areas far from homes and shops, marked the second. The implication of the Plan Chatarra was clear: trash was dirty; dirt bred bugs; bugs carried disease to people; concentrations of trash must also lead to concentrations of dengue. One official emphasized in the conservative daily newspaper *La Prensa* that "chatarreras are sites of large mosquito breeding areas.... [These] businesses have exposed more of the population to...dengue."[1] Patron–client relations were central to the chatarra business as well. Large, well-capitalized chatarra buyers in Managua would routinely sponsor smaller buyers. These smaller buyers, in turn, would work to develop reputations among scavengers as fair-minded and generous in their payouts.

Both the disputes at the dump and the Plan Chatarra reveal how persons and things and creatures that look singular can have multiple identities. The work of collecting and circulating garbage was a mode of *personal* survival that, paradoxically, threatened *population* health. Garbage scavengers were alternately the cause of and the solution to the dengue crisis. The state and the health ministry seemed to be acting both to promote the welfare of the city's poorest residents and to undermine it.

It is certainly not news that some city dwellers, from North Carolina to Nicaragua to Nairobi, survive by scavenging for garbage of value, but from late 2005 until the global financial meltdown of 2008, the world market for recyclables reached unprecedented heights (Medina, 2008). As market prices for recyclables went up, the number of scavengers also increased, and scavengers saw their claims to that material deteriorate rather than improve. From just ten licensed chatarreras in 2005, the city counted 26 by the end of 2008. Scavengers I interviewed in 2008 told me that increased competition during the price boom caused their earnings for an eight-hour workday to drop to a low of just 30 córdobas (roughly $1.50) from a high of more than 100 córdobas. The average adult supported at least three family members.[2] The entanglement of human bodies with mosquitoes and garbage was thus mediated by economic volatility. Just as dengue epidemics can spike rapidly in unexpected places due to circulation of people, viruses, and materials and then recede with little warning, global prices for aluminum, steel, plastics, and paper rise and fall with impressive speed. Over the course of 2008, Nicaragua's garbage trade reached a climax, producing up to 40 million dollars for the national economy.[3] Later that year, in the wake of the global economic crisis, the business crashed. It was during the boom, however, that the protest in the dumps occurred and the Plan Chatarra was put into action.

Garbage, abjection, and conflict

Around 1998, after rains from Hurricane Mitch flooded homes on the shores of Lake Managua, government resettlement plans moved some scavengers to Ciudad Sandino. "We kept scavenging," one scavenger said of the move. "Back then there was lots of garbage coming in, and no one else bothered with it." People had been making a living by scavenging since the opening of Managua's large open-air dump in 1972. (The Nicaraguan term for "garbage scavenger," *churequero*, comes from the nickname for Managua's dump, "La Chureca.") After the hurricane, many of those who had been resettled would pack material from Ciudad Sandino and drive it to Managua, where buyers paid better prices.

Everyone involved in the trade kept up with the prices for different materials, from plastic and paper on the cheaper end to copper and bronze on the higher end. The key to being a good chatarrero and cultivating a base of client churequeros was a reputation not just for prices that matched the accepted daily rate but for fair weights and measures. Churequeros quickly turned on patrons whom they considered dishonest, and chatarreros were careful to inspect sacks of material before payment, looking for rocks and sand hidden within to increase their weight and value.

As these checks and balances developed, a steady supply of waste streamed into Ciudad Sandino. Trucks from nearby apparel factories established in free trade zones (*zonas francas*) carted scrap shoe soles, shredded fabric, and giant plastic packing sacks – all recyclable, all valuable – into the dump. In the early years of the new century, the number of zonas francas was growing. During the same period, municipal solid waste was becoming more saturated with valuable items.

It was at this time that, among Ciudad Sandino's churequeros, a labor organization of sorts emerged – albeit one with no clear leader. The churequeros started to come to the consensus that the city garbage collectors' poaching of the waste stream had become intolerable. When I asked why the scavengers had organized, their answers were framed moral terms. Going into the dump every day and collecting for eight to ten hours was preferable to working on the streets. This hard work, in a recognizable workplace, helped keep people away from drugs and crime. In a city where formal employment was difficult to find, *churequeando* was a morally acceptable alternative to other "underground" methods of making a living. Churequeros did not understand why city leaders should undermine this by allowing city collectors, who already had paying jobs, to scavenge. Churequeros who ventured into the streets to look for chatarra were seen as "delinquents," "thieves," and "vagrants." As either undereducated young people or "older" (i.e., older than 30) adults, churequeros' chances of securing formal employment in places like the zonas francas were small. Churequeros, in other words, were cut out of a new system of trade and work that had allowed cheap, recyclable materials to proliferate in Nicaragua. Recalling the older form of trade and work, they asserted that their work in the dump was a contribution to the city. "Put it this way," one churequero told me: "How would it be if we *didn't* live this way? We'd really be the worst city in Nicaragua."

The city-employed garbage collectors, by contrast, all belonged to an established and powerful labor union, historically dominated by loyalists to the Frente Sandinista de Liberación Nacional (FLSN), the party that led Nicaragua's 1979 left-wing revolution. The FSLN's leader, Daniel Ortega, was elected president in 2006, 16 years after the defeat of the Revolution.

Union activists argued that what churequeros did was not really "work." As Ulrich Schilz, Managua's sanitation supervisor, declared in an editorial published in the normally left-leaning newspaper *El Nuevo Diario*, "The churequeros are not workers; they are informal businesspeople who sell their labor to no one. They exploit themselves, a few with great success.... The only one who gives value to a product is the worker.... In this case, the product is the organization and cleaning of garbage.... The agents of the informal, opportunistic economy don't add any value to this product."[4] From the union's point of view, the churequeros were not working in cooperation with a party or a government. They were parasites, living on the margins of the city. Unionized collectors represented themselves more positively, as underpaid and overworked providers of a "service." The city could never pay them enough in cash for the service they rendered. It owed them the chance to make extra money by recycling.

Yet senses of moral obligation among city collectors were more complex. Don Nelson, a garbage truck driver, confessed in an interview: "I don't really think we should be doing it, and we didn't do it so much before. The churequeros are poor and they live on the garbage. But I...let the others [the *recolectores*, who put garbage into the truck] recycle. They don't earn as much money as I do; they also need the income." Don Nelson was ambivalent about the union's defense of scavenging. As an economic resource, garbage was, at least intuitively, "for" those really in need. The churequeros were precisely the kinds of people that the Sandinista revolution was supposed to bring into the community of citizens. The churequeros were not simply economic adversaries, and the government patrons were not simply distributors of resources.

The dump protests ended in a partial victory for the garbage collectors' union. Each collecting crew, led by a truck driver, negotiated with the churequeros about which materials it would salvage and sell and which it would leave for those in the dump. Even before dengue entered the picture, the politics of chatarra in Ciudad Sandino centered on a set of contradictions. Was waste a collective nuisance or a privatizable resource? Could it be both? If waste was a nuisance or, worse, a threat to public health, what would best control it, state regulation or a more streamlined market? The Plan Chatarra, which went into effect just weeks after the settlement of the dump strike, only piled on the paradoxes.

Plan Chatarra

Chatarreros saw the Plan Chatarra as scapegoating. In a June 2008 meeting at Ciudad Sandino's main health center, they asked repeatedly for "proof" that their businesses were sites of mosquito propagation. "We fumigate," they said. "We have sanitary licenses from the city, from MINSA." "Why this sudden change in the rules?" "How come we are being held responsible *now* if we know dengue affects us every year?"

The health center's director, wielding a dry erase marker, tried to explain the health implications of Nicaragua's garbage economy for his audience. "You see," he began, "there are large brokerages, medium brokerages, and small – we say 'family' – brokerages." He drew parallel horizontal lines on the board to schematically indicate the medium and small brokerages. As he descended, each line became longer, forming a pyramid. Then, below the last line, which indicated the "family" brokerages, he began making vertical, slashing hash marks, indicating that they were more numerous than the large and medium ones. "What's the problem with all these small brokerages? They are inside the barrios, inside the...center of the city." He circled one of his hash marks, making dots around it. "There are houses, businesses, schools." He paused, almost like a preacher or a schoolteacher giving a scolding. "And what happens when an infected mosquito...lives there?" He paused again. Having temporarily silenced the room, he went on to give an extensive recap of the life cycle of the *Ae. aegypti* mosquito, explaining how it might propagate from a chatarrera, the small scale commercial recyclers.

I attended this meeting expecting this sort of interaction: defensiveness from the chatarreros, loquacious scientific speechifying from the MINSA authorities. What I did not expect was the candid appeal to environmental stewardship on the part of the chatarreros that followed. One by one, the chatarreros – mostly men, but a few women – rose to explain to the director that they were "responsible" businesspeople. They were quite aware of the stigma of dealing in garbage, but, they repeated over and over again, "If we did not have this business, where would the garbage go? Who would you blame then?" The chatarreros, they argued, were "cleaning up" the city. Moreover, they were providing "employment." The director's pyramid had yet another rung, even lower and even wider, made up of churequeros, for whom wealthy Nicaraguans had an entomological nickname: *hormigas* (ants), presumably because a churequero carrying a giant sack of empty bottles or cans resembles an ant lugging an improbably large morsel of food.

"Who are our clients?" one man asked, impatiently. "They are the old, the children, the most poor. If you move us out of the city, where will they go? Are you going to ask an old man to walk five, six kilometers out of town so he can survive? This is their survival!" The brokers were styling themselves less as sanitary citizens than as responsible patrons.

To Don Eliseo Ordoñez, it was not surprising that MINSA launched the Plan Chatarra when it did, in April 2008. Don Eliseo was the owner of one of Nicaragua's four largest chatarreros, a patron to many small family chatarreros, and a leader in the Association of Recyclers of Nicaragua (Asociación de Recicladores de Nicaragua, or ASORENIC). His business was one of collection and export. He bought aluminum, plastic, paper, and assorted metals in bulk, loaded them onto shipping containers, and sent them abroad. The destinations of these shipments tended to be in Asia, particularly China, where a boom in construction meant high demand for cheap raw material. Don Eliseo was politically and socially active. Among other things, he had been involved in the years before Ortega and the FSLN returned to power with an effort to lobby the Association of Nicaraguan Municipalities to replace municipal garbage collection services with private firms such as his. Starting in 2002, ASORENIC began to style itself as a pro-environment, pro-health organization. That year, it generated a press release promoting the recycling business as a way to connect Managua to a globalizing world, asking, "If they can do it in Miami, in Los Angeles, in Mexico, in Guatemala, in Costa Rica, or in any other country in the world, why NOT in NICARAGUA?" When the Ministry of Health initiated the Plan Chatarra, ASORENIC again began making the case that the private sector – not the state – could best handle urban sanitation. The firms would pay the cities for the right to collect valuable garbage and profit by selling the vastly increased volume they would yield. Given that projects like the rebuilding of Ciudad Sandino's infrastructure in the days after Hurricane Mitch relied upon private enterprise, such a proposal might not have seemed so far-fetched.

Don Eliseo had no doubt that MINSA had hatched the Plan Chatarra as a response to a political opportunity created by the churequeros' protests. The protests had been covered extensively in the national television and print media, and Managua's dump, "La Chureca," was already a high-profile stain on the government's reputation. It was the largest open-air waste facility in Central America, and it had become a regular tour stop for photographers and non-government organization (NGO) activists looking either to expose environmental damage and extreme poverty. Ciudad Sandino's "chureca" was a similar if less well-known site. Located just a few steps away from a large, private charity health clinic, Ciudad Sandino's dump was also regularly visited by foreign volunteer and aid groups. Given the proliferation of painful images of dumps and their inhabitants on television, the Internet, and in newspapers, Don Eliseo explained, Ortega's new FSLN government was under pressure to do something. The protests against city garbage collectors who seemed to be skimming resources from their needy residents could not have come at a worse time. They had further undermined the public's trust in city services.

As a result of the protests, Don Eliseo told me, "the government realized how lucrative the business is, and they are setting up these restrictions on us so that they can take it over." To Don Eliseo, the Plan Chatarra was nothing more than parasitism. The government was using the pretense of dengue to disrupt a long-standing and productive set of reciprocal patron–client relationships that linked large buyers like himself to street-level churequeros. For the business-minded leaders of ASORENIC, the solution to the health problems posed by garbage was not a crackdown on scavenging but a formalization of it. Such a formalization would modernize Nicaragua, improve health, and, presumably, allow private businesses to handle a problem that the corrupt state was clearly ill equipped to address. When the Plan Chatarra was put into action, "family" chatarreros cited their role in "cleaning" the city and giving the poorest of the poor a chance to make a living. Large chatarreros like Don Eliseo took this narrative of environmental stewardship one step further, playing on the struggles of the poor and trumpeting the market to frame the garbage trade as a "comedy of the commons," in which harvesting waste seemed like a solution to, rather than a symptom of, the ravages of poverty (Hardin, 1968; Rose, 1986).

Don Eliseo's suspicions about a vast state conspiracy notwithstanding, in mid-2008, Ciudad Sandino and the rest of Managua *were* facing the onset of another dengue epidemic, and traders *were* seeing record highs in the prices of recyclable materials. The number of chatarreras and churequeros *was* swelling, it seemed, alongside the number of dengue cases. The correlation between this market surge and the epidemic surge was circumstantial rather than causal, but it had power nonetheless.

There is little doubt that the spaces where garbage changes from waste to commodity sometimes overlap with the spaces where mosquitoes reproduce and spread disease. Mosquitoes, therefore, actively mediated the conflict of economic and environmental management that was occurring at the height of Ciudad Sandino's garbage boom. Waste and mosquitoes "explained each other" (Robbins, 2012, p. 95). City garbage collection services, however partial, depended on the idea that the solution to environmental problems began in homes. For residents who had access to regular curbside pickup, a failure to dump signaled a glaring absence of social responsibility – of sanitary citizenship. Those who insisted on harboring garbage in their homes were named and shamed by their neighbors. A similar discourse surrounded the management of mosquitoes. Mosquitoes were a public problem that originated in private space. People who refused to have their homes purged of insects faced public rebuke. In the more marginal barrios where scavengers resided, however, the division of space and responsibility into stark categories of public and private did not make as much sense. Houses in these areas were much more tenuously private. Many churequeros had constructed their homes out of donated material, on land they did not own. Others were deep in debt to private electrical and water companies. Churequeros who had no legal title to their own houses showed me power bills that reached into the tens of thousands of *córdobas*. In the face of aggressive bill collectors, house abandonments were a fairly common occurrence. Residents thus had trouble seeing the upkeep of their homes as a long-term private interest, much less a public one.

The idea that dengue "hot spots" can be localized by identifying "high-risk" zones like chatarreras or the homes of churequeros is more easily postulated than proven (Adams & Kapan, 2009). *Ae. aegypti* are highly adapted to human movements, breed in small colonies, and are difficult to isolate. In addition, most dengue cases are asymptomatic. Absent a massive sample of human blood for evidence of latent dengue antibodies, there was no practical way that MINSA could have proven that hot spots existed around chatarreros. The Plan Chatarra raised pressing questions about how to regulate a disease with no cure or effective prophylactic, in an environment where overcoming poverty often trumped other collective priorities, including health and sanitation.

Moral economy of mosquito control

The Plan Chatarra linked the recycling business to disease, but it was more than the fact that chatarreros traded in garbage that bothered MINSA officials. After all, as Don Eliseo and other chatarreros reminded me, "We are helping to clean up Nicaragua."

The problem was the manner in which they traded. More insidious still, as was noted both in published press accounts and in the June meeting between the director of Ciudad Sandino's health center and the local brokers, was the proximity of "small," "family" recycling brokerages to private homes.[5] Chatarreros were bad neighbors. Still, MINSA's efforts to regulate them failed to change the system just as completely as did the churequeros' efforts to secure rights to scavenge. That failure stemmed in part from the sheer ambition of the Plan Chatarra. Ending garbage scavenging once and for all would have been nearly impossible. The plan did nevertheless strain the relationship of "client" chatarreros to large "patron" brokers like Don Eliseo.

In early summer 2008, the small chatarreros of Ciudad Sandino learned that an advocacy alliance was being formed. An environmental NGO that also claimed to represent banana plantation workers injured by the pesticide Nemagon was being financed by ASORENIC, the consortium of Managua's largest garbage brokers, to organize opposition to the Plan Chatarra. By paying a membership fee to the NGO, Ciudad Sandino's chatarreros would receive a card that identified them as "recyclers," along with a small diploma, and a blue-green, earth-themed sticker to place on their front doors. The sticker read, WE THE CHATARREROS OF NICARAGUA DEMAND THAT THE GOVERNMENT RESPECT US AND ALLOW US TO WORK FOR THE DAILY BREAD OF OUR CHILDREN. GOD BLESS THIS NATION. YES TO WORK! NO TO UNEMPLOYMENT! Like the churequeros, these normally independent actors would band together, making a moral case for their rights to collect and sell waste.

Doña Nubia was one of the first to join. She opened up a chatarrera in her small house near the main entrance to Ciudad Sandino around 2007. She had lived there since the 1980s, when the revolutionary government gave her land as compensation for her husband's death in an industrial accident. For most of her life, she had been a street vendor, selling juices and flavored ice at the bus stop near the barrio's entrance. As she got older, that work became a strain on her knees and back, and her son, who owned a small pickup truck, suggested that she begin work as a chatarrera. Doña Nubia's chatarrera was typical of the cottage industry that blossomed and withered in the space of a few short "boom" years in the late 2000s. Her main tool was a heavy-duty scale, of the kind that was common in meat or grain stalls in Managua's markets. It was a bronze, spring-calibrated mechanism with a sharp hook attached to one end and an eye attached to the other. Doña Nubia had it nailed to a rafter overhanging her small front porch. On a large piece of scrap roofing metal, her son had fashioned a sign in black paint that read SE COMPRA CHATARRA. Churequeros, local schoolchildren, and neighbors would arrive with sacks of plastic, aluminum, steel, copper, or other items (usually presorted), and Doña Nubia would weigh them and pay a per-pound rate, which she set by taking a small reduction from the rate she would receive from a larger buyer in Managua. Then she would empty the bag into one of the larger piles of like materials that dotted her patio. When the piles became large enough (or the price spiked high enough), her son would load them into the pickup and sell them to a trusted patron.

Like most of the 26 other chatarreros in Ciudad Sandino, Doña Nubia was visited by representatives of ASORENIC's environmental NGO, who convinced her to pay and join. As they explained, dengue was a danger, but the real problem was that the government was overregulating the garbage, a nuisance to be sure, but also an "inexhaustible resource." If they would let the chatarreros treat it for what it was, health and wealth would both improve. During our interview at his office, Don Eliseo showed me a PowerPoint presentation he had prepared for municipal governments interested in privatizing their garbage services. Its concluding slide contained green words on a gray background: *Basura=$* (Garbage equals money). As one of his own business circulars noted, "Chatarra represents a great source of income, not just for its owner, but for the country, if we just take advantage of it." Don Eliseo was linking the commoditization of garbage to the achievement of health and wealth. MINSA's renewed zeal for regulating recycling, he insisted, had little to do with health.

This, as it turned out, wasn't Don Eliseo's first fight against the health ministry. ASORENIC had been confronted by MINSA in 2002 over accusations that the industry's dependence on informal collection networks was bad for public health. That year, ASORENIC sent MINSA an open letter, portraying chatarreros as a group of petty patrons, "Recycling businesspeople, the vast majority of whom are humble, honest, hardworking people, have found a way to make a living, improve their economic situation, and PROVIDE WORK TO THOUSANDS OF NICARAGUANS." In 2002, MINSA and the rest of the Nicaraguan government were run by a largely pro-business, center-right regime. This message had a supply-side tint that was missing from the "bottom-up" flavor of the 2008 response to MINSA sanctions. The 2008 response was built not around talk of trickle-down economics but around the colorful, earth-themed environmental logo. Though the environmental alliance ASORENIC formed was shaky, the quick organization of patron and client chatarreros against MINSA proved somewhat effective. The literally and metaphorically "green" logo started popping up on the walls of chatarreros all around town.

Then September came, and everything changed. The bottom fell out of the scrap metal industry, as the global financial crisis slowed world trade to a crawl. Indeed, in the words of Hilario Zepeda, a chatarrero who was elected to Ciudad Sandino's municipal council on the FSLN ticket earlier in 2008, once the prices went down and the churequeros' dump protests were out of the news, MINSA seemed to forget about them. But he and every other chatarrero I met in Ciudad Sandino also reported that ASORENIC and the environmental NGO had also disappeared. "I think [the NGO] just wanted us to pay our inscription fees, to buy our little ID cards and be done with us," said Doña Nubia, whose business failed to survive the price crash. "They won't be back. MINSA won't be back."

Doña Lesbia, a chatarrera who lived in Zona 8, concurred. In hindsight, she couldn't understand why the NGO identification card said "recycler" and not "chatarrera." Recycling seemed like the act of a conscientious consumer, not a trader. She didn't think of herself in any particular way as an environmentalist. The truth was, "chatarra is a dirty thing. It's something that dirties you." A younger woman with little experience in the trade, Doña Lesbia was approached by a large buyer in Managua who wanted to make an inroad in Zona 8. He loaned her a scale and taught her about how to weigh and value copper, aluminum, bronze, steel, and plastic. When the crash ended her relationship with that patron, she, like Doña Nubia, had to diversify. When I met her, she was in the process of starting a door-to-door tortilla business. She kept the "recycler" sticker on the wall of her patio (she liked its bright colors), but as a small chatarrera, she no longer mattered, either as an object of state scrutiny or as a symbol of "sustainable" capitalism.

Doña Lesbia's ambivalence about being called a "recycler" was telling. Perhaps she was aware of her status as a vulnerable "middle person," a parasitic figure in a pyramid scheme dominated by large interests like Don Eliseo's. She had come to see what other churequeros were seeing: in a commoditized landscape, the kinds of rights a poor person could assert – including the rights that come with clientage – began to shrink (Purcell, 2002). Recycling was part of a survival strategy, but it was hard to turn it into a civic action. "Rights" to collect were not given.

MINSA lacked the power to convince people in greater Managua that the junk business as it was – an open range where technological, political, and monetary might determined who had resource rights – might be dangerous enough to public health to be regulated. The more garbage circulated, the less it seemed to be a common concern. Or perhaps Don Eliseo was onto something – perhaps the Ortega government wanted to add chatarra to the list of industries in which it had a major stake and from which it could provide a lucrative outlet for loyalists.[6] In an ecological sense, mosquitoes and the virus had taken advantage of the situation, thriving in a set of spaces (dumps, streets, parks, and gutters) that were neither public nor private, neither common nor collective.

"Dirtiness," as Doña Lesbia reminded me, was "part of the business."

Patrons, clients, and parasites

The last time we spoke, shortly before she closed the chatarrera, Doña Nubia told me the story of how her neighbor's child was stricken with dengue. "The child got sick, and soon MINSA and the neighbors were coming here telling me that the mosquitoes came from me." She paused. "Do you think that's possible?" she asked. "That a mosquito from here made her sick? There are clouds of mosquitoes in Ciudad Sandino."

She paused again and looked pensively in the direction of her neighbors' house. Neighborhood FSLN activists eager to carry out the Plan Chatarra had fueled the accusation that the child's sickness was her fault. "They'll be happy now because now I'm not buying anything anymore." She threw her hands up in the direction of the last pile of scrap metal in the corner of her porch. By the time of our last conversation, in November 2008, few people were coming by to sell chatarra. In any case, Doña Nubia could rarely afford to buy it, given the depth to which prices had fallen. So the material sat there, rusting and collecting the last of the seasonal rains. And Doña Nubia sat beside it, pondering the lives of mosquitoes, of the little girl – now, thankfully, fully recovered from her bout with dengue – and of rumors from her fellow chatarreros about the prospect of a market recovery: a recovery that might make her solvent once again, but might also, once again, make her the object of neighborly and state scorn.

In the Plan Chatarra, it was small operators like Doña Nubia who received the bulk of MINSA's attention. In an anti-dengue crusade built on a hygienic premise, that clean homes harbored few mosquitoes while "dirty" ones were potential breeding spots, this made perfect sense. It also made sense that the connection between chatarra and dengue became strongest when the market was strongest. Intuitively, it would appear that a strong market for recyclables *could* produce a cleaner and maybe even "healthier" city. What better incentive to clean than money? Yet the market could do little to produce a sense of ethical or social connection. Indeed, combined with a mounting series of dengue epidemics, the growth in the garbage market actually turned certain spaces and the bodies that occupied them into dangerous internal threats. Along the way, it destabilized the patron–client system that regulated the circulation of garbage. Under stable circumstances, chatarreros and churequeros, even as "dirty workers," could rightfully claim to be improving public space. The soaring market, however, brought the details of the trade to broader attention. All of a sudden, churequeros and chatarreros appeared dangerously unconcerned with the quality of private spaces: of their own homes and bodies. It was their seeming disregard for the interior worlds they shared with mosquitoes that made them suitable objects of scorn.

The churequeros and chatarreros certainly made easy targets as public health officials in Nicaragua searched for someone to blame for the ever-mounting number of dengue cases. Scavenging disrupts standard narratives about the proper relationship between people and the things they buy, sell, and consume. People tend to characterize waste as polluting and dangerous, and turning it into value seems to violate basic norms about the proper way to make a living (see Douglas, 2002 [1966]; Moore, 2008). The economic lives of the chatarrero and the churequero seem somehow "parasitic." These actors thrive by milking the dark underside of a larger system of trade and consumption.

In another sense, however, chatarreros and churequeros were themselves beset by parasites. As clients, the churequeros and chatarreros of Ciudad Sandino depended upon the buying power of large patrons in Managua and beyond. Chatarreros and churequeros provided cheap, free labor for these well-capitalized entities, as well as for the city planners who – whether they openly admitted it or not – depended upon an army of *hormigas* to keep the streets minimally clean. The assignment of blame rested not only on ideas about the ethics of seeking profit from the waste that was so prominent in the urban landscape but also on normative ideas about ecology. The spaces that brigadistas and MINSA officials called *focos* (or what English-speaking entomologists sometimes call mosquito "hot spots"), from piles of garbage to flower pots, were essential for the reproduction of life in the city. The mosquito, too, seemed to behave in a parasitic fashion, feeding and breeding opportunistically among humans in these same spots.

Parasitic relationships tend to complement and build upon one another. It is impossible to disaggregate the parasitic relationships between scavengers and large brokers from those between mosquitoes and people. Householders in poor cities cannot survive without scavenging. The global consumer economy arguably cannot thrive without the work of informal scavengers. Mosquitoes cannot spread without the help of the human garbage trade. Mosquitoes and garbage do something more than make people sick; they are productive of political and social relationships.

Seeing human and insect lives as entangled makes it difficult to argue that a will to sanitary citizenship – the kind of will that mosquito control programs are meant to instill – inevitably results from membership in a "consumer society." One of the lessons of both studies of parasitic relations in nature and those of patron–client relations in Latin American social life is that the terms of such relations are interchangeable. Beyond anthropocentrism, there is no necessary reason to see viruses or mosquitoes (both of which are much more abundant on Earth than are human beings) as thriving parasitically upon humans. It seems just as reasonable to say that epidemics of dengue, avian influenza, and the like are the result of *human* parasitism: exploitation of global resources, excess consumption, global warming, and the like. Likewise, in the patron–client relationship, who is behaving parasitically and who is being preyed upon depends upon one's point of view. Are garbage scavengers milking the city's material excess, or is the city milking the labor of scavengers to keep those excesses out of sight and out of mind? Power resides among those who can identify and neutralize parasites and clients.

Philosopher Michel Serres (2007 [1982]) argues that parasitic relations – relations of disruption and disturbance – are the norm rather than an exception in social life. For global health, the parasite is a device for thinking of the ways in which environments are inhabited – constantly made and unmade – rather than simply occupied. While this volume is dedicated to exploring "resistance" in global health, parasitism might be a productive alternative. In Nicaragua, a local manifestation of a global health policy (dengue mosquito control) disrupted a local economy, but the reverse was also the case. Parasitism emphasizes multidirectional "noise" over binary acts of domination and resistance. In Nicaragua, a local conflict masked the global contradiction that increased consumption of disposable goods, even among the poor, makes parasites of almost everyone. Cities, and certain groups within them, become both reviled for their association with waste and indispensable to the reproduction of the economy.

In Nicaragua, parasitism happened at both a material and a symbolic level. At the material level, the fact that dengue mosquitoes could potentially find a harbor in otherwise valuable waste made these wastes even more abject. At a symbolic level, the circulation of wastes and mosquitoes through urban space – private, public, collective, and in between – altered the social meanings of those spaces. From a free-market point of view, for-profit recycling might be seen as a cure to the environmental ravages of urban life, and the chatarrera might be a site of a kind of "green capitalism," while from MINSA's point of view, the same space could be one of risk and danger, or a threat to social solidarity. The connections between waste and dengue are far from direct, but neither are those between scavenging and sustainability. The absence of clear rights, whether those of churequeros to make a living from the dump, of the city government to regulate and resell refuse in the name of the public interest, or of MINSA to make the health implications of the postconsumer economy a point of public consideration, ultimately benefited large operators like Don Eliseo – and small ones, like *Ae. aegypti*.

Editor commentary

Alex Nading suggests that we reconsider concepts of parasitism and its relationship to established systems. He argues:

- Parasitism provides a conceptual framework to recognize that environments are inhabited rather than occupied, and that the relationship between humans and the environment is multidirectional.
- Humans as consumers of disposable goods are as much parasites as mosquitoes and the dengue virus they carry.
- *Sanitary citizenship* implies will and agency, introduced by institutions in power and enforced by communities through local interpretations of morality and moral behavior as a public good.
- Community participation through economic opportunities (i.e., the commoditization of garbage) can improve public health, possibly in more ways than disease-specific health interventions.
- Disturbance and disruptions are norms rather than exceptions in social life.

Notes

1 *La Prensa*, August 4, 2008.
2 These data are based on a survey I conducted while interviewing adult (older than 16 years) churequeros in 2008 (n=50).
3 *El Nuevo Diario*, October 14, 2008.
4 *El Nuevo Diario*, March 24, 2008.
5 *La Prensa*, August 7, 2008; *El Nuevo Diario*, July 24, 2008.
6 *El Nuevo Diario*, September 29, 2009.

References

Adams, B., & Kapan, D. D. (2009). Man bites mosquito: Understanding the contribution of human movement to vector-borne disease dynamics. *PLoS One*, *4*(8), e6763. doi:10.1371/journal.pone.0006763

Ashencaenen-Crabtree, S., Wong, C., & Mas'ud, F. (2001). Community participatory approaches to dengue in Sarawak, Malaysia. *Human Organization*, *60*(3), 201–208.

Beck, U. (1992). *Risk Society: Towards a New Modernity*. London: Sage.

Briggs, C. L., & Mantini-Briggs, C. (2003). *Stories in the Time of Cholera: Racial Profiling during a Medical Nightmare*. Berkeley: University of California Press.

Carter, E. (2012). *Enemy in the Blood: Malaria, Environment, and Development in Argentina*. Tuscaloosa: University of Alabama Press.

Douglas, M. (2002 [1966]). *Purity and Danger: An Analysis of Concepts of Pollution and Taboo.* London: Routledge.

Gubler, D. J. (1989). *Aedes aegypti* and *Aedes aegypti*–borne disease control in the 1990s: Top down or bottom up. Charles Franklin Craig Lecture. *American Journal of Tropical Medicine and Hygiene, 40*(6), 571–578.

Hardin, G. (1968). The tragedy of the commons. The population problem has no technical solution; it requires a fundamental extension in morality. *Science, 162*(3859), 1243–1248.

Hartmann, C. D. (2012). Uneven urban spaces: Accessing trash in Managua, Nicaragua. *Journal of Latin American Geography, 11*(1), 143–163.

Medina, M. (2008). The Informal Recycling Sector in Developing Countries: Organizing Waste Pickers to Enhance Their Impact. *Gridlines: Sharing Knowledge, Experiences, and Innovation in Public-Private Partnerships in Infrastructure. Note 44* (pp. 1–4).

Moore, S. (2008). The politics of garbage in Oaxaca, Mexico. *Society and Natural Resources, 21*(7), 597–610.

Nading, A. (2012). "Dengue mosquitoes are single mothers": Biopolitics meets ecological aesthetics in Nicaraguan health work. *Cultural Anthropology, 27*(4), 572–596.

Nading, A. (2014). *Mosquito Trails: Ecology, Health, and the Politics of Entanglement.* Oakland: University of California Press.

Peterson, A., & Lupton, D. (1996). *The New Public Health: Health and Self in the Age of Risk.* London: Sage.

Purcell, M. (2002). Excavating Lefebvre: The right to the city and its urban politics of the inhabitant. *GeoJournal, 58*(2–3), 99–108.

Robbins, P. (2012). *Political Ecology: A Critical Introduction* (2nd ed.). New York: Blackwell.

Rose, C. (1986). The comedy of the commons: Custom, commerce, and inherently public property. *The University of Chicago Law Review, 53*(3), 711–781.

Serres, M. (2007 [1982]). *The Parasite* (L. R. Schehr, Trans.). Minneapolis: University of Minnesota Press.

Standish K., Kuan G., Avilés W., Balmaseda A., & Harris E. (2010). High dengue case capture rate in four years of a cohort study in Nicaragua compared to national surveillance data. *PLOS Neglected Tropical Diseases*, 4(3), e633.

5

WHEN NEW SCIENCE MEETS OLD TRADITIONS

Engaging the Indigenous Sector to Improve Uptake of Voluntary Medical Male Circumcision for HIV Prevention in High-Prevalence Countries

Nicola Bulled and Edward C. Green

An association between male circumcision (MC) and HIV infection was first recognized in the late 1980s (Bongaarts, Reining, Way, & Conant, 1989; Moses et al., 1990). Yet, geographic correlations and ecologic case/control and cohort studies from around the world were inconclusive in establishing a clear causal relationship.[1] What appeared to be beneficial in some areas and among some communities, proved ineffective or even increased risk of infection in others. In their review of the growing literature on MC by Brian Morris and Xavier Castellsague (2011) suggest that MC does have substantial benefits in reducing HIV infectivity, both directly and via syndemic relationships with other sexually transmitted infections. For its simplicity, voluntary male medical circumcision (VMMC) is an alluring HIV prevention strategy. The procedure requires only minimal engagement with the health system, as compared to long-term HIV treatment regimens, and does not require consistent negotiations of risk reduction, as is the case with condom use and reduced sexual partnerships. In an effort to spur action, the scientific community determined that unprecedented, gold standard RCT clinical studies should be initiated to ascertain the medical value of MC and settle the debate.[2]

The independently conducted RCTs from South Africa (Auvert et al., 2005), Kenya (Bailey et al., 2007), and Uganda (Gray et al., 2007) each identified an almost 60% reduction in HIV infection risk among circumcised men. Based on these findings, mathematical models suggest that VMMC can reduce HIV incidence by at least 1% per year, with a relative reduction in prevalence of 25 to 67% in different populations after accounting for the average duration of HIV disease (Gray et al., 2003; Nagelkerke, Moses, de Vlas, & Bailey, 2007; Orroth et al., 2007; Williams et al., 2006). Should these results hold in the general population, then as Wamai and colleagues stated, "There is no biomedical intervention currently being implemented that has been demonstrated *scientifically* to be more efficacious or cost-effective than male circumcision" (2012, p. 118, emphasis added).

Although RCTs estimate the effectiveness of VMMC within controlled settings, non-clinical/study data has left some doubt regarding the value of VMMC in reducing HIV incidence. For example, data collected via national demographic and health surveys (DHS) from large representative population samples in 19 African countries suggest no difference in HIV prevalence (measured by blood samples) by circumcision status (*self-reported*) (Garenne, 2008, 2010; Mishra, Hong, & Khan 2006; Way, Mishra, & Hong, 2006). Two countries have significantly lower HIV prevalence among circumcised men (Kenya and Uganda), while three countries (Lesotho, Malawi, and Tanzania) have higher levels of HIV infection among circumcised men. In Lesotho, HIV prevalence is higher in circumcised men: 21 compared to 16% (MoHSW, 2009). DHS data from Swaziland in the mid-2000s also indicated a greater risk of HIV infection among circumcised men: 22 compared to 20% (MoEPD, 2008). A more recent Swaziland HIV Incidence Measurement Survey found that circumcised men are statistically less likely to be HIV infected (16.4 compared to 25%; $p<.001$, SHIMS, 2014).

By 2007, rising concerns over the ineffectiveness of efforts to control the HIV pandemic (Dowsett & Couch, 2007), as well as the limited success and slow progress of other potential prevention technologies (e.g., microbicides, vaccines, and pre-exposure prophylactics), compelled the World Health Organization (WHO) to officially endorsed VMMC as a cost-effective HIV prevention approach (WHO/UNAIDS, 2007). The official statement from WHO came after a conference of experts in Montreux, Switzerland, which included academic researchers, members of international health organizations, gender relations specialists, representatives of UN funding agencies and of other public and private institutions, association members, youth organization members, and human rights activists. In addition, 16 representatives from Member States and 11 from civil society, including women's health advocates and a representative from the Global Network of People Living with HIV, were invited to present their interpretations and perspectives on the issue (UNAIDS, 2007). While a range of stakeholders were involved in this effort to exchange views and discuss the consequences of VMMC, much of the meeting program focused discussions on the *science* of VMMC. Little time was dedicated to discussing implementation, ethics (human rights), or the findings from studies being conducted by the Social Aspects for HIV/AIDS Research Alliance group (Dowsett & Couch, 2007; Garenne, Giami, & Perrey, 2013).

For many, the global policy on VMMC was established too hastily and in a manner that left little room for voicing dissent, and it overly valued scientific evidence with limited concern for context. Gary Dowsett, the sole critic of VMMC in attendance at the Montreux conference, and his colleague Murray Couch (2007, p. 43) have positioned these considerations in terms of epistemology and politics: "What is at stake, how is that defined and by whom, what evidence suffices, who decides and on what basis?" Kirsten Bell (2015, p. 2) has suggested that VMMC was essentially "made into the 'right' tool for the job of reducing HIV transmission," given the ineffectiveness of all other current strategies[3] and the desire to find some new and potentially effective approach to addressing HIV.

In this chapter, we compare responses to the global VMMC initiative in two small southern African countries – Lesotho and Swaziland. These two countries are particularly instructive, as their realities contradict the evidence upon which global VMMC policy was established – both countries have heavy HIV burdens but contrasting MC practices. Swaziland is currently recognized as having the highest prevalence of adult HIV/AIDS in the world (31%) (Bicego et al., 2013), with Lesotho in second place (22.9%) (UNAIDS, 2013b).

However, Lesotho and Swaziland have contrasting legacies of MC. In Lesotho, MC traditionally occurs during *lebollo*, a rite of passage undertaken by adolescent boys involving tests of physical and mental fortitude (including circumcision) to mark the transition to manhood. Neonatal circumcision is uncommon, as is circumcision during adolescence/adulthood in a biomedical facility – that is, until recent VMMC initiatives to prevent HIV took effect. Traditional circumcision has been on the decline, especially among men in urban areas who, driven by new economies that value education and formal labor, can neither find the time for, nor see the value in, such a practice (MoH, 2014). Latest estimates indicates that 77% of Basotho men over the age of 15 are circumcised: 49% traditionally circumcised, 28% medically circumcised, and 5% both traditionally and medically circumcised (MoH, 2014). The secretive nature of the practice and frequent newspaper articles from South Africa, where similar cultural practices have become more dangerous, resulting in deaths and penile amputations (Apps, 2005; Malan, 2013; Nandipha, 2013), have heightened fears and dissuaded participation in traditional circumcision. Furthermore, returning boys are often considered dangerous, unruly, and defiant (Bulled, 2015b). The result is a type of embodied class division (Aggleton, 2007). Swaziland does not have a recent history of practicing MC, either as part of puberty rites ceremonies or as a biomedical procedure on neonates or adults; most recent surveys estimate that between 16% and 20% of Swazi men are circumcised (Adams & Moyer, 2015; SHIMS, 2014). Neither Swaziland nor Lesotho were quick to respond to the VMMC agenda, with hesitance expressed at the levels of national government, traditional leadership, and the individual.

MC cannot completely explain the HIV epidemics in Lesotho and Swaziland. A complex interplay of behavioral, social, economic, historic, and political factors contribute to HIV burdens. Many of these factors likely overlap, given Swaziland and Lesotho's geographies and relationships with shared neighbor South Africa. But the situation does allow for an interesting backdrop upon which to base some theoretical questions. If mathematical models based on RCT results are accurate, why are there not significant differences in HIV prevalence between Lesotho and Swaziland?[4] How do resource-limited nation-states respond to global calls to action when their own realities, and readings of the evidence, appear to contradict interpretations offered by those with global authority? In this light, we focus this chapter on exploring the hesitance offered towards global public health VMMC agendas and through this reveal the inherent inequities in current global public health architecture and propose a new way forward.

We are not arguing for or against the VMMC strategy. As practitioners who have both worked on HIV prevention programming, we strongly believe that prevention efforts of all kinds must continue. Global interests and funding for new approaches, or a reinvigoration of old strategies, is waning. Integrating technologies into risk prevention may provide both the stimulation and the solutions needed. Our aim in this chapter is not to suggest that VMMC is not one of these useful strategies. Rather, we wish to highlight that true and genuine collaboration is imperative to successfully develop and integrate such solutions.

Introducing, making medical, and re-medicalizing male circumcision

MC has historically been practiced, forgotten and practiced again. In the U.S. and the U.K., MC fell out of favor given limited scientific evidence of its value. Despite a strong opposition movement in the 1960s, MC was re-medicalized in the U.S. as a common procedure in neonates. By contrast, in the U.K., analyses revealing little population benefit at high cost to the National Health System significantly reduced the number of neonatal circumcisions performed (Carpenter, 2010). The association between HIV and MC has in some places reignited a fading medical practice, established a new medical practice, or made medical what was once a social ritual, often associated with religious identity.

Following WHO's announcement in support of VMMC, 14 countries in the AIDS belt of southern Africa, including Lesotho, were identified as priority areas for VMMC programs to address the HIV epidemic. However, in the 2013 UNAIDS Global Report, Lesotho, along with four other countries where VMMC was stated to be a priority (Malawi, Namibia, Rwanda and Zimbabwe), coverage of VMMC for adults had achieved less than 10% of the targeted number (UNAIDS, 2013a). Despite the endorsement of the global authority on disease policies, some at-risk populations, governments, and academics have not willingly accepted the VMMC approach. Indeed the promotion and implementation of VMMC is proving much harder than donors and health experts anticipated. Emmanuel Njeuhmeli, Senior Biomedical Prevention Advisor in the USAID Office of HIV/AIDS, assessing VMMC as an HIV prevention strategy, notes that "we have reached only one-third of the 20.3 million interventions [VMMC procedures] needed to achieve maximum public health benefit by the end of 2016" (MacDonald & Njeuhmeli, 2014). Reasons for this low VMMC uptake in resource-poor settings include barriers to service delivery, such as limited infrastructure (surgical theatres and surgeons required by some health authorities, including the Ministry of Health in Lesotho) and resource constraints (stock-outs of essential circumcision commodities).

The WHO also notes that progress in the universal promotion of VMMC has been constrained due to "*uncertain client demand*" (WHO, 2013, p. 6). PEPFAR has acknowledged that overcoming limited demand has proven considerably more difficult than addressing supply-side barriers (USAID, 2013). In a review of initial acceptability studies conducted in nine countries in sub-Saharan Africa, VMMC was generally recognized as a suitable practice for disease prevention (Westercamp & Bailey, 2007). The median proportion of uncircumcised men willing to become circumcised was 65%

(range: 29–87%). Women generally favored circumcision of their partners (47–79%) and were willing to circumcise their sons (70–90%). However, other studies indicate greater variation in acceptability of the practice. Most Xhosa men in a peri-urban area of Cape Town, South Africa, a community that practices traditional MC, were unwilling to undergo VMMC or allow their sons to do (Mark et al., 2012). Despite being aware of the HIV preventive benefits that VMMC may provide, community members argue that they already practice MC and do so in a way that honors their own cultural identities and notions of manhood (Mark et al., 2012). A study in Malawi found that acceptability varied based on prior experience with or historical practices of MC, with greater acceptance in districts where MC was practiced (Ngalande, Levy, Kapondo, & Bailey, 2006). These variations in acceptability highlight the complexity of social meanings that are attached to MC (Aggleton, 2007; Garenne et al., 2013; Gollaher, 2000; Vincent, 2008a); indeed, "being circumcised involves deep-seated values, beliefs, and motivational factors that vary with ethnic, religious, and cultural identities" (Njeuhmeli quoted in MacDonald & Njeuhmeli, 2014).

Lesotho: Medicalizing MC

An initial rapid assessment and cost-effectiveness analysis was conducted in 2007 in Lesotho, following the WHO endorsement of VMMC, with a full situational analysis completed in 2008 (MoHSW, 2008). Results indicated a minimum VMMC population coverage of 52% to evoke significant impact on reducing HIV prevalence or close to 35,000 procedures performed in 2009 and 44,000 annually thereafter (NAC, 2010). Provision of VMMC would have to increase by a factor of seven in order to meet this target. For such a scale-up, an annual investment of 1.2 million USD was deemed necessary. The projected impact was estimated as one averted HIV infection for every 6.1 surgeries conducted. Two-thirds of health centers reported not having the capacity required by the national government to perform VMMC surgeries, and most would need significant facility upgrades and trained health-care personnel. At the time, guidelines, protocols, site assessment, monitoring and evaluation tools, and a counselling package were identified as close to finalized (NAC, 2010). Nine hospitals were assessed and equipment and consumables procured to support the scale-up plan.

In 2009, a year after finalizing the VMMC initiation plan, a Lesotho national newspaper headline read, *Health Ministry has no intention of campaigning for circumcision.* The title of this article was misleading, as then Director General of Health, Dr. Mpolai Moteetee, was specifically referencing neonatal circumcision, stating that "circumcising young children . . . is against the Basotho culture" (Linake, 2009, p. 8). Even so, while remarking about the association found between VMMC and HIV infection, he made no mention of government support of VMMC in Basotho adolescents or adult men. Official government efforts to fully initiate VMMC services were delayed until 2012, six years after the WHO formally endorsed the strategy and two years after the national plan was finalized. At this time, the Ministry of Health aimed to reach 80% coverage by 2017, or 317,215 men age 15–49 years.

The hesitance to initiate a complete national VMMC program is multifaceted. First, there is the lack of a clear relationship between MC and HIV among Basotho men. The Lesotho DHS from 2004 and 2009 articulate this:

> The relationship between male circumcision and HIV levels in Lesotho *does not conform to the expected pattern of higher prevalence among uncircumcised men*. HIV prevalence is substantially higher among circumcised men age 15–59. . . . Moreover, the pattern of higher HIV prevalence among circumcised men is the same across a large majority of subgroups. (MoHSW, 2009, p. 212, emphasis added)

The more recent 2014 DHS makes no mention of the association, even though data were collected on both HIV and MC status. Instead the 2014 DHS references a study conducted on Lesotho Defense Force recruits that identified incomplete MC among those who reported being circumcised (Thomas et al., 2011). Incomplete circumcision may not provide the same level of protection from HIV (Fahrbach, Barry, Anderson, & Hope, 2010; Morris & Wamai, 2012). Surprisingly, incomplete circumcisions were identified in both men who reported traditional (72%) and those reporting biomedical (27%) procedures. The presence of Langerhans cells within the foreskin allows for the internationalization and transport of HIV. At high viral loads Langerin (contained within Langerhans cells) is unable to clear the virus, resulting in systemic infection (Morris & Castellsagué, 2011). Without the foreskin, Langerhans cells cannot internalize the virus.

Second, while not officially referenced by Ministry of Health representatives, traditional leaders in charge of organizing and maintaining cultural rites, including *lebollo*, expressed concern over the VMMC agenda and the transfer of MC to biomedical venues (Bulled, 2013). In addition, according to the Lesotho Ministry of Health and Social Welfare, suggestions to implement standardized certification requirements for all traditional healers/circumcisers, in an effort to more closely monitor *lebollo* circumcision practices, have not been well received by indigenous leadership (Linake, 2010).[5] Although these approaches aim to ensure effective practices, there are concerns that opening up traditional MC procedures to outside medical scrutiny risks disclosing deep ritual secrets to outsiders and the consequent weakening of the power of the rite of passage.[6]

Finally, given the extent of *lebollo* engagement, supporting an approach that appears anti-cultural or unsupportive of Basotho identity requires care. The global VMMC agenda hit Lesotho at a time of political transition, when politicians were vying for votes from constituents in both rural and urban areas. Ultimately, government leaders opted to simply consider scientific/biomedical methodologies and resulting data to evaluate the applicability of global VMMC directives for the local situation.

While not officially recognized by the government as part of the coordinated national efforts, VMMC surgeries have been offered since 2007, when a male clinic was established in Lesotho's capital city, Maseru, run by the Lesotho Planned

Parenthood Association. Here, reportedly 240 men, ages 17 and up, undergo VMMC every month (Matope, 2010). VMMC procedures are also performed in government health facilities, hospitals, filter clinics, and private surgeries, at a cost that varies from 6 to 74 USD. A national assessment of MC published in 2008 estimated that approximately 4,000 to 6,000 VMMC are performed each year (MoHSW, 2008). Beginning in 2012, international organizations (funded by PEPFAR, with the operational assistance of Jhpiego, an international nonprofit organization affiliated with Johns Hopkins University) provided six international medical doctors to perform VMMC procedures.[7] The non-governmental organization, Population Services International, also launched VMMC efforts in collaboration with the Lesotho Defense Force.[8] These international agents operating locally supported VMMC taking place only in modern biomedical facilities. By implication, this support indicated opposition towards the unsafe and improper traditional circumcisions that take place at *lebollo* initiation schools (Vincent, 2008b, p. 81).

Swaziland: Introducing a new practice

Given that MC has not been routinely practiced in Swaziland since the time of King Mswati II (Marwick, 1940), MC for HIV prevention purposes had to be officially reintroduced. The 2006 DHS noted that the relationship between MC status and HIV infection was not consistent with RCT findings, but offered that "the relationship between male circumcision and HIV infection may be confounded by the fact that the circumcision may not involve the full removal of the foreskin" (MoEPD, 2008, p. 235). Encouraged by the VMMC movement and external donors, the government of Swaziland introduced a national VMMC policy in 2007. While this policy aimed to make VMMC services available to men of all ages, the scale-up of services targeted primarily HIV-negative men ages 15–24 and neonates. To stimulate greater movement towards VMMC, PEPFAR funded an ambitious plan in 2010 to rapidly circumcise 80% of Swazi males. The program was implemented through a partnership between the Ministry of Health and Social Welfare and the U.S.-based Futures Group. The program was called the Accelerated Saturation Initiative (ASI) and was known in siSwati as *Soka Uncobe*, which carries the double meaning of 'circumcise' and 'conquer' (Adams & Moyer, 2015). Two years later, only 20% of the targeted boys and men of Swaziland were reached, at a cost of 484 USD per circumcised male (Adams & Moyer, 2015; Masinga, 2012; MoH, 2012).

A number of factors contributed to the failure of the ambitious scale-up program. First, the ASI felt imposed from the outside, with King Mswati II "roped in[to]" the VMMC issue. Approval and buy-in from the king was necessary to initiate the project, but locals felt he was pushed into supporting VMMC as a universal practice for men by foreigners rather than of his own accord. Second, free VMMC services generated suspicion, linking what was perceived as an externally imposed biomedical intervention to the numerous HIV conspiracy theories that circulate in the region (Kalichman, 2009; Stadler, 2003). Both factors contributed to overall uncertainty and confusion, as noted by Mabuza of NERCHA (Swazi National AIDS Committee): "There were a lot of issues involving male circumcision that were not properly explained to Swazi men, so they rejected it and they talked to their friends, and word of mouth was negative instead of positive" (IRIN, 2013).

Negative word of mouth has prevented many men in Swaziland from circumcising. A survey commissioned by the Futures Group in 2011 found that there was 91% awareness of circumcision nationally. However, in the mid-2000s only four in ten uncircumcised men indicated an interest in being circumcised (MoEPD, 2008). Pain (52%), physical changes involved (11%), tradition/religion and continued belief in witchcraft (10%), fear (6%), older age (6%), and a general lack of understanding of the procedure are all factors inhibiting individual engagement in VMMC (Adams & Moyer, 2015; MoEPD, 2008).

The widespread and continued belief in witchcraft also proved an unanticipated barrier to ASI's promotions of VMMC. Health Minister Xaba alluded to this when he told the *Times of Swaziland*, "Some men feared that the foreskin could end up in wrong hands, being used by some unscrupulous people for their ulterior motives" (IRIN, 2013). Criminals are known to seek strengthening potions made with human body parts. Victims, usually children or older people, are found with organs and other body parts missing, with genitalia highly sought after. Consequently, the uncertain endpoint of the removed foreskin is of grave concern for men contemplating VMMC procedures; as noted by one young Swazi man, "That's also what I wanted to know and they wouldn't tell me – what happens to my foreskin once it is cut off?" The program director of a faith-based HIV initiative in Manzini explained,

> It would have been easy to be honest and explain to the Swazi men that their foreskins would be incinerated like all surgical refuse. But the promoters said, 'Oh, no, we can't talk about witchcraft. What will the donors say?'. . . [Consequently] the circumcision initiative failed because of arrogance on the part of its promoters.

Finally, there was uncertainty regarding the continued need to practice safe sex following surgery. Many young men noted that if they still needed to use condoms, what was the purpose of the procedure? A university student, Samkelo, commented, "When I heard I would still have to wear a condom, I said, 'What is the point?'" These statements suggest that individuals and officials consider multiple and various rational factors when contemplating the painful VMMC procedure.

Implications

The varying acceptability and the limited effect of VMMC in reducing population prevalence of HIV highlight the importance of the policy development process and the inclusion of key stakeholders in the development of policy, interventions, and messages of persuasion. In the development of the official WHO/UNAIDS VMMC policy, the involvement of key stakeholders was limited. Specifically, while community members and people living with HIV were invited to attend the Montreux conference of 'experts,' traditional healers/circumcisers, who have had a long-standing stake in the discussion of MC, were left out of the conversation (Garenne et al., 2013). Traditional healers in southern Africa were fundamental in identifying the relationship between MC and lower HIV and sexually transmitted infection rates early on in the epidemic (Green, 1994, 2000). The WHO/UNAIDS statement provided no space for considering the role that these and other stakeholders have in developing and shaping VMMC strategies (Bulled, 2015a).

To not consider the role that indigenous leaders or traditional healers/circumcisers may have in the conversation regarding MC limits the likely effectiveness of the strategy to adapt to highly mobile patterns of social change, including integration of biomedical strategies, rapidly changing sexual cultures, and markers of identity (Aggleton, 2007; Dowsett & Couch, 2007). Furthermore, the VMMC policy anticipates that individuals will act upon the scientific evidence with limited concern for alternative justification, practices, or barriers to action. Only recently, given the lower-than-anticipated uptake and impact of the VMMC approach, have serious conversations surfaced that suggest different messages are needed to address varying social groups and their unique concerns (Brooks et al., 2010; Gilliam et al., 2010; Sgaier, Reed, Thomas, & Njeuhmeli, 2014).

Echoing the sentiments of Bell (2015), we suggest that an expansion beyond the either/or scenarios of VMMC/MC a greater consideration for alternatives to parameters that alter the current bureaucratic, imposed, top-down approaches of global health delivery are necessary. We have suggested more direct and equitable engagement with indigenous leaders and traditional healers as partners in VMMC efforts in order to take greater advantage of their important social positions (Bulled & Green, 2015). Such collaborations have been attempted with various ethnic groups in South Africa. Training programs specifically implemented in the Eastern Cape Province (among the Xhosa and Pondo) have successfully shown that traditional healers/circumcisers can be trained to improve their knowledge of HIV prevention strategies and attitudes towards collaborations with biomedical health-care providers, consequently adopting safer and more effective MC strategies (Kanta, 2004; Peltzer, Nqeketo, Petros, & Kanta, 2008). In Lesotho, the general and progressive decline in participation in rites of passage provide a possible opening for programs interested in 'upgrading' traditional MC practices. Chiefs and ceremonial elders also expressed an interest and need for training and education to bring them up-to-date on issues related to HIV and sexual health. Traditional leaders and members of the Council of Initiators view this training approach as empowering, as it ensures that (1) an important cultural practice is maintained; (2) practices of traditional healers do not contribute to the transmission of HIV; and (3) traditional circumcisers will perform a service that offers some protection to the people of Lesotho, based on available evidence (Bulled, 2013).

Alternatively, there have been attempts to integrate VMMC procedures conducted by biomedical providers within initiation rites. In some communities in Zimbabwe (Harmon, 2011), South Africa (Vincent, 2008b), and Kenya

(WHO, 2009), where traditional MC is performed, the initiates schedule VMMC surgeries immediately prior to embarking on their rites; or, male medical doctors and nurses attend the initiation ceremonies to conduct the circumcision. In this way the initiates receive safe, sterile, and complete surgeries that are integrated within the traditional rites practice. While effective, both this approach and the implementation of standardized national regulations[9] limit and jeopardize the practices of traditional healers/circumcisers and threaten to devalue their role in their communities (Vincent, 2008b). Vincent argues that traditional healers/circumcisers/leaders resist the intrusion of state influence into their domain, as these individuals have limited marketable skills and opportunities for the assertion of power or status (Vincent, 2008b). Consequently, 'tradition' is viewed as a limited currency with which to trade for power, and one that state regulations and biomedical intrusion risk further devaluing.

A possible alternative to extensive regulations or the integration of VMMC procedures by biomedical providers into traditional ceremonies is the implementation of new devices that have been developed that might prove useful in non-surgical contexts. For example, the PrePex and Shang Ring employ radial elastic pressure, causing distal necrosis for easier removal of the foreskin (Barone et al., 2011; Kigozi et al., 2013; Mutabazi et al., 2013). The non-surgical VMMC approach takes significantly less time than surgical methods; does not require injections or sterile settings; is bloodless; has been deemed safe; and seems suitable for nurses, health workers, and trained traditional circumcisers or healers to conduct (Bitega, Ngeruka, Hategekimana, Asiimwe, & Binagwaho, 2011; Mutabazi et al., 2012).

Reconfiguring the global health architecture

The case of VMMC as a new HIV prevention strategy presents itself as a global endeavor – an interconnectedness of ideas, interpretations, and reflexivity across national borders and geographical and ideological boundaries (Guill´en, 2001; Robinson, 2001; Tomlinson, 1999). The RCTs, cost-effectiveness, and acceptability studies assessing VMMC for HIV prevention were conducted in the global South. Yet, the studies' conceptualization, organization, and funding were developed in the global North. Following on this globally interconnected trend, in a concerted effort to ignore (social) boundaries in setting the global policy on VMMC, the WHO and UNAIDS convened the Montreux conference, inviting a diverse group of interdisciplinary participants from the global North and South. However, Western biomedical ideologies predominated, with the results of the RCTs considered more valid than discussions on how these scientific findings might be interpreted (or implemented) in diverse social contexts (Dowsett & Couch, 2007).

Consequently, despite gestures to appear to obtain multiple perspectives, the VMMC agenda of global health institutions is heavily influenced by Western-based biomedical ideologies of the global North, founded on scientific claims of truth. The invited community members served as mere token representatives in the global discussions (Dutta, 2011), with little opportunity provided to consider the diverse concerns and realities of those seeming to stand the most to gain. Continued debates raised over the translation of biological effectiveness into effective public health interventions, given highly varied geopolitical and cultural context (Boyle & Hill, 2011; de Camargo, de Oliveira Mendonça, Perrey, & Giami, 2013), are touted as anti-scientific, or "reject[ing] established scientific norms and rules, so making scientific discourse all by impossible" (Wamai et al., 2012, p. 119). However, as argued by Harry Marks, the presumed truth of scientific efforts have relevance only in spreadsheets and controlled settings, losing their meaning when integrated into reality (including theoretical and empirical literature) (cited in Epstein, 1996, p. 197). The current VMMC/MC debate is oddly reminiscent of the academic/activists disputes that occurred during the uncertain periods of HIV discovery and later treatment (Epstein, 1996). In this, the comments made by Merrill Singer in 1994 (p. 1323) reflect the global responses to epidemic HIV of both the past and the present: "The AIDS text is multivocal, and includes not only the voice of authority but also the voice of resistance."

The HIV pandemic has already shown that in order for prevention and treatment approaches to prove successful, collaboration, integration, and new ways of thinking are necessary. Medical professionals, governments, and donors need to overcome any prejudices against collaborating with non-biomedical representatives, in this case members of the indigenous sector, a sector which is routinely ignored, circumvented, or condemned by the modern sector. Concurrently, traditional healers/circumcisers and others who operate in and represent the indigenous sector (e.g., chiefs, spiritual leaders, and other ritual specialists) would have to agree to *change* what might be considered a crucial element in a centuries-old rite of passage endorsed by ancestral spirits (in groups that practice MC), or agree to promote the approach (in groups that do not practice MC).

While hesitance of individuals to engage with and nation-states to adopt the global VMMC agenda is regarded as non-compliance, the cases of Swaziland and Lesotho indicate a resistance to assumptions of *homogeneity* of HIV epidemics and the behavioral, social, economic, historical, political, and cultural conditions that drive the epidemics; the *universal applicability* of Western biomedical approaches; and the continued *inequitable structures of global health governance*. Furthermore, in employing scientific discourse, pointing to national health statistics, and indicating that rational action to prevent disease does not need to involve surgery, expertise is asserted and a shared position of authority within current global public health structures negotiated.

Editor commentary

In this chapter, Bulled and Green have offered an interpretation of why the update of a new HIV prevention technology, VMMC, has been slower than anticipated by leaders in global HIV/AIDS governing bodies despite a shared global desperation to find new HIV prevention strategies. Looking specifically at the situations in Lesotho and Swaziland, where HIV burdens are similar but engagement with MC is distinct, resistance to the global agenda highlights the continued need to do the following:

- Consider diverse disease contexts and the unique intersections of the factors influencing disease burdens
- Recognize the inappropriateness of considering universal applications of biomedical strategies to address disease
- Address the inequity that exists in global health governance structures that allows certain voices to be considered superior, certain data to be considered more valid, and certain conditions to be considered a greater need

Notes

1 Geographical correlations suggested a negative relationship between HIV disease and circumcision practices in Africa, with lower HIV prevalence in Sahelian West Africa, where MC is more uniformly conducted, as compared to Eastern Africa, where circumcision is less routinely practiced (Bongaarts, Reining, Way, & Conant, 1989; Moses et al., 1990). Ecological case/control and cohort studies revealed a less conclusive relationship. While appearing to hold in some countries in Africa, this was not the case in all countries (Bongaarts et al., 1989; Drain, Halperin, Hughes, Klausner, & Bailey, 2006; Halperin & Bailey, 1999; Moses et al., 1990; Siegfried et al., 2005; Weiss et al., 2008; Weiss, Quigley, & Hayes, 2000). Many studies indicate that throughout Europe, the U.S., New Zealand, and Australia MC has no effect on STIs transmitted either through homosexual or heterosexual routes (Dave et al., 2003; Dickson, van Roode, Herbison, & Paul, 2008; Laumann, Masi, & Zuckermann, 1997; Richters, Smith, de Visser, Grulich, & Rissel, 2006). However, a systematic review and meta-analysis indicates that MC does reduce risk of some STIs in certain populations (Morris & Castellsagué, 2011; Weiss, Thomas, Munabi, & Hayes, 2006).

2 For a detailed overview of the historical debate on the medical value of MC, see David Gollaher's (2000) book *Circumcision: A History of the World's Most Controversial Surgery*.

3 The view of Edward C. Green (author) is that primary prevention was never really tried, only risk reduction, based on the belief that sexual behavior cannot be changed much. Breaking up multiple concurrent partner sexual networks was/is considered "sex-negative" and non-supportive by the risk-reduction industry.

4 At present, there is insufficient data to determine if incomplete MC contributes to this apparent anomaly, or what effect reaching sexual debut prior to MC may have on national data.

5 Nkonyana, J. (2012, 18 October). Ministry of Health and Social Welfare, HIV/AIDS. Personal communication with N. Bulled.

6 Dlamini, M. (2014, 6 February). Prince of Swaziland Royal Family. Personal communication with E.C. Green. This is often the first, or formal reaction to a proposal framed this way. With the right, respectful approach, what might be perceived or articulated as "cultural barriers" can be overcome.

7 Koppenhaver, T. (2012). USAID/PEPFAR. Personal communication with N. Bulled. Nkonyana, J. (2012, 18 October). Ministry of Health and Social Welfare, HIV/AIDS. Personal communication with N. Bulled.

8 Pedersen, B. (2011). Population Services International, Technical Services Advisor. Personal communication with N. Bulled. Walto, D. (2011). Population Services International/Lesotho Director. Personal communication with N. Bulled.

9 The Application of Health Standards in Traditional Circumcision Act No. 6 of 2001 regulates traditional initiation practices in South Africa (SAPA, 2013).

References

Adams, A., & Moyer, E. (2015). Sex is never the same: Men's perspectives on refusing circumcision from an in-depth qualitative study in Kwaluseni, Swaziland. *Global Public Health*, 1–18. doi:10.1080/17441692.2015.1004356

Aggleton, P. (2007). "Just a Snip"?: A social history of male circumcision. *Reproductive Health Matters*, *15*(29), 15–21.

Apps, P. (2005, 28 July). Deaths Prompt Action on Circumcision Schools. *Reuters/IOL*.

Auvert, B., Taljaard, D., Lagarde, E., Sobngwi-Tambekou, J., Sitta, R., & Puren, A. (2005). Randomized, controlled intervention trial of male circumcision for reduction of HIV infection risk: The ANRS 1265 Trial. *PLoS Medicine*, *2*(11), e298.

Bailey, R. C., Moses, S., Parker, C. B., Agot, K., Maclean, I., Krieger, J. N., . . . Ndinya-Achola, J. O. (2007). Male circumcision for HIV prevention in young men in Kisumu, Kenya: A randomised controlled trial. *Lancet*, *369*(9562), 643–656.

Barone, M. A., Ndede, F., Li, P. S., Masson, P., Awori, Q., Okech, J., . . . Goldstein, M. (2011). The Shang Ring device for adult male circumcision: A proof of concept study in Kenya. *Journal of Acquired Immune Deficiency Syndromes*, *57*(1), e7–12.

Bell K. (2015). HIV prevention: Making male circumcision the 'right' tool for the job. *Global Public Health*, *10*(5–6), 552–72.

Bicego, G. T., Nkambule, R., Peterson, I., Reed, J., Donnell, D., Ginindza, H., . . . Justman, J. (2013). Recent patterns in population-based HIV prevalence in Swaziland. *PLoS One*, *8*(10), e77101. doi:10.1371/journal.pone.0077101

Bitega, J. P., Ngeruka, M. L., Hategekimana, T., Asiimwe, A., & Binagwaho, A. (2011). Safety and efficacy of the PrePex device for rapid scale-up of male circumcision for HIV prevention in resource-limited settings. *Journal of Acquired Immune Deficiency Syndromes*, *58*(5), e27–134.

Bongaarts, J., Reining, P., Way, P., & Conant, F. (1989). The relationship between male circumcision and HIV infection in African population. *AIDS*, *3*(6), 373–377.

Boyle, G., & Hill, G. (2011). Sub-Saharan African randomized clinical trials into male circumcision and HIV transmission: Methodological, ethical and legal concerns. *Journal of Law and Medicine*, *19*(2), 316–334.

Brooks, R., Etzel, M., Klosinski, L., Leibowitz, A., Sawires, S., Szekeres, G., . . . Coates, T. (2010). Male circumcision and HIV prevention: Looking to the future. *AIDS and Behavior*, *14*(5), 1203–1206. doi:10.1007/s10461-009-9523-4

Bulled, N. (2013). New lives for old: Modernity, biomedicine, traditional culture and HIV prevention in Lesotho. *Global Discourse*, *3*(2), 284–299.

Bulled, N. (2015a). Hesitance towards voluntary medical male circumcision in Lesotho: Reconfiguring global health governance. *Global Public Health*, *10*(5–6), 757–772. doi:10.1080/17441692.2014.962559

Bulled, N. (2015b). *Prescribing HIV Prevention: Bringing Culture into Global Health Communication.* Walnut Creek, CA: Left Coast Press.

Bulled, N., & Green, E. C. (2015). Making voluntary medical male circumcision a viable HIV prevention strategy in high-prevalence countries by engaging the traditional sector. *Critical Public Health*, *26*(3), 258–268. doi:10.1080/09581596.2015.1055319

Carpenter, L. M. (2010). On remedicalisation: Male circumcision in the United States and Great Britain. *Sociol Health Illn*, *32*(4), 613–630. doi:10.1111/j.1467-9566.2009.01233.x

Dave, S., Johnson, A., Fenton, K., Mercer, C., Erens, B., & Wellings, K. (2003). Male circumcision in Britain: Findings from a national probability sample survey. *Sexually Transmitted Infections, 79*, 499–500.

de Camargo, K. R., de Oliveira Mendonça, A. L., Perrey, C., & Giami, A. (2013). Male circumcision and HIV: A controversy study on facts and values. *Global Public Health, 8*(7), 769–783.

Dickson, N., van Roode, T., Herbison, P., & Paul, C. (2008). Circumcision and risk of sexually transmitted infections in a birth cohort. *Journal of Pediatrics, 152*(3), 383–387.

Dowsett, G.W., & Couch, M. (2007). Male circumcision and HIV prevention: Is there really enough of the right kind of evidence? *Reproductive Health Matters, 15*(29), 33–44.

Drain, P. K., Halperin, D.T., Hughes, J. P., Klausner, J. D., & Bailey, R. C. (2006). Male circumcision, religion, and infectious diseases: An ecologic analysis of 118 developing countries. *BMC Infectious Diseases, 6*, 172.

Dutta, M. J. (2011). *Communicating Social Change: Structure, Culture, and Agency*. New York, NY: Taylor & Francis.

Epstein, S. (1996). *Impure Science: AIDS, Activism, and the Politics of Knowledge*. Berkeley, CA: University of California Press.

Fahrbach, K. M., Barry, S. M., Anderson, M. R., & Hope, T. J. (2010). Enhanced cellular responses and environmental sampling within inner foreskin explants: Implications for the foreskin's role in HIV transmission. *Mucosal Immunology, 3*(4), 410–418. doi:10.1038/mi.2010.18

Garenne, M. (2008). Long-term population effect of male circumcision in generalized HIV epidemics in sub-Saharan Africa. *African Journal of AIDS Research*, 7(1), 1–8.

Garenne, M. (2010). Mass campaigns of male circumcision for HIV control in Africa: Clinical efficacy, population effectiveness, political issues. In G. Denniston, F. Hodges, & M. Milos (Eds.), *Genital Autonomy: Protecting Personal Choice* (pp. 49–60). Dordrecth: Springer Science & Business Media B.V.

Garenne, M., Giami, A., & Perrey, C. (2013). Male circumcision and HIV control in Africa: Questioning scientific evidence and the decision-making process. In T. Giles-Vernick & J. L. Webb Jr. (Eds.), *Global Health in Africa: Historical Perspectives on Disease Control* (pp. 185–210). Athens: Ohio University Press.

Gilliam, F., Brooks, R., Leibowitz, A., Klosinski, L., Sawires, S., Szekeres, G., . . . Coates, T. (2010). Framing male circumcision to promote its adoption in different settings. *AIDS and Behavior, 14*(5), 1207–1211. doi:10.1007/s10461-009-9656-5

Gollaher, D. L. (2000). *Circumcision: A History of the World's Most Controversial Surgery*. New York, NY: Basic Books.

Gray, R. H., Kigozi, G., Serwadda, D., Makumbi, F., Watya, S., Nalugoda, F., . . . Wawer, M. J. (2007). Male circumcision for HIV prevention in men in Rakai, Uganda: A randomised trial. *Lancet, 369*(9562), 657–666.

Gray, R. H., Li, X., Wawer, M. J., Gange, S. J., Serwadda, D., Sewankambo, N. K., . . . Group, T. R. P. (2003). Stochastic simulation of the impact of antiretroviral therapy and HIV vaccines on HIV transmission: Rakai, Uganda. *AIDS, 17*(13), 1941–1951.

Green, E. (1994). *AIDS and STDs in Africa: Bridging the Gap between Traditional Healers and Modern Medicine*. Boulder, CO: Westview Press.

Green, E. (2000). Male circumcision and HIV infection (Letter). *The Lancet, 355*(9207), 926–927.

Guill´en, M. (2001). Is globalization civilizing, destructive or feeble? A critique of five key debates in the social science literature. *Annual Review of Sociology, 27*, 235–260.

Halperin, D., & Bailey, R. C. (1999). Male circumcision and HIV infection: Ten years and counting. *Lancet, 354*(9192), 1813–1815.

Harmon, K. (2011). Can male circumcision stem the AIDS epidemic in Africa? *Scientific American*. Retrieved from http://www.scientificamerican.com/article.cfm?id=male-circumcision-hiv-epidemic&page=3.

IRIN. (2013). Circumcision plans go awry in Swaziland. Retrieved from www.irinnews.org/printreport.aspx?reportid=98023

Kalichman, S. (2009). *Denying AIDS: Conspiracy Theories, Pseudoscience and Human Tragedy*. New York, NY: Copernicus Books.

Kanta, X. (2004). *Traditional Male Circumcision and Intitiation into Manhood: Legal, Health and Environmental Perspectives*. Gonubie, Eastern Cape: Impilo ya Bantu Health and Development Projects.

Kigozi, G., Musoke, R., Watya, S., KSighoma, N., Ssebbowa, P., Serwadda, D., . . . Gray, R. (2013). The acceptability and safety of the Shang Ring for adult male circumcision in Rakai, Uganda. *Journal of Acquired Immune Deficiency Syndromes, 63*(5), 617–621.

Laumann, E., Masi, C., & Zuckermann, E. (1997). Circumcision in the United States. Prevalence, prophylactic effects and sexual practice. *Journal of the American Medical Association, 277*(13), 1052–1057.

Linake, M. (2009, July 13). Health ministry has no intentions of campaigning for circumcision. *Informative*, p. 8.

Linake, M. (2010, 26 October). Male circumcision crucial in reducing chances of HIV infection. *Informative*. Retrieved from http://www.informativenews.co.ls/index.php/archives/2420-male-circumcision-crucial-in-reducing-chances-of-hiv-infections-

MacDonald, R., & Njeuhmeli, E. (2014). Assessing voluntary medical male circumcision for HIV prevention in a unprecendented public health intervention. *PLOS Collections, 2014* (May 7).

Malan, M. (2013, August 16). The boys who lost their manhood. *Mail & Guardian*. Retrieved from http://mg.co.za/article/2013-08-16-00-the-boys-who-lost-their-manhood

Mark, D., Middelkoop, K., Black, S., Roux, S., Fleurs, L., Wood, R., & Bekker, L.-G. (2012). Low acceptability of medical male circumcision as an HIV/AIDS prevention intervention within a South African community that practises traditional circumcision. *South African Medical Journal, 102*(6), 571–573.

Marwick, B. (1940). *The Swazi*. London: Frank Cass & Co.

Masinga, W. (2012, 10 January). Over 34000 men circumcised. *Swazi Observer*. Retrieved from http://www.observer.org.sz/index.php?news=34135

Matope, T. (2010, 18 October). Men throng clinic for circumcision. *Public Eye*. Retrieved from http://www.publiceyenews.com/2010/10/18/men-throng-clinic-for-circumcision/

Mishra, V., Hong, R., & Khan, S. (2006). Risk behaviors and patterns of HIV seroprevalence in countries with generalised epidemics: Results from the demographic and health surveys. Paper presented at the XVI International AIDS Conference, Toronto, Canada.

MoEPD. (2008). *Swaziland Demographic and Health Survey 2006–2007*. Mbabane, Swaziland: Ministry of Economic Planning and Development, Central Statistical Office, Macro International Inc. Retrieved from http://www.measuredhs.com/pubs/pdf/FR202/FR202.pdf

MoH. (2012). *Quarterly Service Coverage Report*. Mbabane: Swaziland Ministry of Health.

MoH. (2014). *Lesotho Demographic and Health Survey 2014, Key Indicators Report*. Retrieved from Maseru: https://www.dhsprogram.com/pubs/pdf/PR62/PR62.pdf

MoHSW. (2008). *Situation analysis report: Male circumcision in Lesotho*. Maseru, Lesotho: Ministry of Health and Social Welfare.

MoHSW. (2009). *Lesotho Demographic and Health Survey 2009*. Maseru, Lesotho: Ministry of Health and Social Welfare, Bureau of Statistics, ORC Macro. Retrieved from http://www.measuredhs.com/pubs/pdf/FR171/FR171-LS04OneLgFile.pdf

Morris, B. J., & Castellsagué, X. (2011). The role of circumcistion in preventing STIs. In G. Gross & S. Tyring (Eds.), *Sexually Transmitted Infections and Sexually Transmitted Diseases* (pp. 715–739). Berlin: Springer.

Morris, B. J., & Wamai, R. G. (2012). Biological basis for the protective effect conferred by male circumcision against HIV infection. *International Journal of STD & AIDS, 23*(3), 153–159.

Moses, S., Bradley, J. E., Nagelkerke, N. J., Ronald, A. R., Ndinya-Achola, J. O., & Plummer, F. A. (1990). Geographical patterns of male circumcision practices in Africa: Association with HIV seroprevalence. *Internationl Journal of Epidemiology, 19*(3), 693–697.

Mutabazi, V., Kaplan, S. A., Rwamasirabo, E., Bitega, J. P., Ngeruka, M. L., Savio, D., . . . Binagwaho, A. (2012). HIV prevention: Male circumcision comparison between a nonsurgical device to a surgical technique in resource-limited settings: A prospective, randomized, nonmasked trial. *Journal of Acquired Immune Deficiency Syndromes, 61*(1), 49–55.

Mutabazi, V., Kaplan, S. A., Rwamasirabo, E., Bitega, J. P., Ngeruka, M. L., Savio, D., . . . Binagwaho, A. (2013). One-arm, open-label, prospective, cohort field study to assess the safety and efficacy of the PrePex device for scale-up of non-surgical circumcision when performed by nurses in resource-limited settings for HIV prevention. *Journal of Acquired Immune Deficiency Syndromes, 63*(3), 315–322.

NAC. (2010). UNGASS country report: Lesotho. January 2008–December 2009. Maseru, Lesotho: National AIDS Commission.

Nagelkerke, N. J., Moses, S., de Vlas, S. J., & Bailey, R. C. (2007). Modelling the public health impact of male circumcision for HIV prevention in high prevalence areas in Africa. *BMC Infectious Diseases*, 7, 16.

Nandipha, K. (2013). Murder charges for botched circumcisions in Eastern Cape. *Mail & Guardian*. Retrieved from mg.co.za/article/2013-07-08-murder-charges-for-botched-circumcisions-in-eastern-cape

Ngalande, R. C., Levy, J., Kapondo, C. P., & Bailey, R. C. (2006). Acceptability of male circumcision for prevention of HIV infection in Malawi. *AIDS Behav, 10*(4), 377–385. doi:10.1007/s10461-006-9076-8

Orroth, K. K., Freeman, E. E., Bakker, R., Buve, A., Glynn, J. R., Boily, M. C., . . . Hayes, R. J. (2007). Understanding the differences between contrasting HIV epidemics in east and west Africa: Results from a simulation model of the Four Cities Study. *Sexually Transmitted Infections, 83*(Suppl 1), 15–16.

Peltzer, K., Nqeketo, A., Petros, G., & Kanta, X. (2008). Evaluation of a safer male circumcision training programme for traditional surgeons and nurses in the Eastern Cape, South Africa. *African Journal of Traditional, Complementary and Alternative Medicines, 5*(4), 346–354.

Richters, J., Smith, A., de Visser, R., Grulich, A., & Rissel, C. (2006). Circumcision in Australia: Prevalence and effects on sexual health. *International Journal of STD and AIDS, 17*(8), 547–554.

Robinson, W. (2001). Social theory and globalization: The rise of a transnational state. *Theory and Society, 30*(2), 157–200.

SAPA. (2013, 10 July). ANCYL: Initiation schools should be regulated. *Mail & Guardian*. Retrieved from http://mg.co.za/article/2013-07-10-ancyl-modern-and-safe-initiation-schools-the-way-to-go

Sgaier, S. K., Reed, J. B., Thomas, A., & Njeuhmeli, E. (2014). Achieving the HIV prevention impact of voluntary medical male circumcision: Lessons and challenges for managing programs. *PLoS Medicine, 11*(5), e1001641. doi:10.1371/journal.pmed.1001641

SHIMS. (2014). Swaziland HIV incidence measurement survey (SHIMS), Results update October 2014: Male Circumcision. Retrieved from http://shims.icap.columbia.edu/key-findings/male-circumcision/

Siegfried, N., Muller, M., Deeks, J., Volmink, J., Egger, M., Low, N., . . . Williamson, P. (2005). HIV and male circumcision: A systematic review with assessment of the quality of studies. *Lancet Infectious Diseases, 5*, 165–173.
Singer, M. (1994). The politics of AIDS: Introduction. *Social Science and Medicine, 38*(10), 1321–1324.
Stadler, J. (2003). Rumour, gossip and blame: Implications for HIV/AIDS prevention in the South African lowveld. *AIDS Education and Prevention, 15*(4), 357–368.
Thomas, A. G., Tran, B. R., Cranston, M., Brown, M. C., Kumar, R., & Tlelai, M. (2011). Voluntary medical male circumcision: A cross-sectional study comparing circumcision self-report and physical examination findings in Lesotho. *PLoS One, 6*(11), e27561.
Tomlinson, J. (1999). *Globalization and Culture.* Cambridge, MA: Polity Press.
UNAIDS. (2007). International experts review male circumcision. Retrieved from http://www.unaids.org/en/resources/presscentre/featurestories/2007/march/20070307mcpt4/
UNAIDS. (2013a). Global Report: UNAIDS Report on the Global AIDS Epidemic 2013. Geneva, Switzerland: Joint United Nations Programme on HIV/AIDS.
UNAIDS. (2013b). Lesotho: HIV and AIDS Estimates (2013). Retrieved from http://www.unaids.org/en/regionscountries/countries/lesotho/
USAID. (2013). Strengthening High Impact Interventions for an AIDS-Free Generation Worldwide (RFA-OAA-14-000001). Retrieved from www.devex.com/projects/grants/strengthening-high-impact-inverventions-for-an-aids-free-generation-worldwide/3736
Vincent, L. (2008a). 'Boys will be boys': Traditional Xhosa male circumcision, HIV and sexual socialisation in contemporary South Africa. *Culture, Health & Sexuality, 10*(5), 431–446.
Vincent, L. (2008b). Cutting tradition: The political regulation of traditional circumcision rites in South Africa's liberal democratic order. *Journal of Southern African Studies, 34*(1), 77–91.
Wamai, R. G., Morris, B. J., Waskett, J. H., Green, E. C., Banerjee, J., Bailey, R. C., . . . Hankins, C. A. (2012). Criticisms of African trials fail to withstand scrutiny: Male circumcision does prevent HIV infection. *Journal of Law and Medicine, 20*(1), 93–123.
Way, A., Mishra, V., & Hong, K. (2006). *Is male circumcision protective of HIV infection? Poster exhibition.* Paper presented at the XVI International AIDS Conference, Toronto, Canada
Weiss, H. A., Halperin, D., Bailey, R. C., Hayes, R. J., Schmid, G., & Hankins, C. A. (2008). Male circumcision for HIV prevention: From evidence to action? *AIDS, 22*(5), 567–574.
Weiss, H. A., Quigley, M. A., & Hayes, R. J. (2000). Male circumcision and risk of HIV infection in sub-Saharan Africa: A systematic review and meta-analysis. *AIDS, 14*(15), 2361–2370.
Weiss, H. A., Thomas, S. L., Munabi, S. K., & Hayes, R. J. (2006). Male circumcision and risk of syphilis, chancroid, and genital herpes: A systematic review and meta-analysis. *Sex Transm Infect, 82*(2), 101–109; discussion 110. doi:10.1136/sti.2005.017442
Westercamp, N., & Bailey, R. C. (2007). Acceptability of male circumcision for prevention of HIV/AIDS in sub-Saharan Africa: A review. *AIDS and Behavior, 11*(3), 341–355.
WHO. (2009). *Traditional male circumcision among young people: A public health perspective in the context of HIV prevention.* Geneva, Switzerland: World Health Organization.
WHO. (2013). *Guideline on the use of devices for adult male circumcision for HIV prevention.* Geneva: World Health Organization Retrieved from http://apps.who.int/iris/bitstream/10665/93178/1/9789241506267_eng.pdf.
WHO/UNAIDS. (2007). *New Data on Male Circumcision and HIV Prevention: Policy and Programme Implications. WHO/UNAIDS Technical Consultation Male Circumcision and HIV Prevention: Research Implications for Policy and Programming Montreux*, 6–8 March. Geneva: World Health Organization and UNAIDS Retrieved from www.who.int/hiv/mediacentre/MCrecommendations_en.pdf.
Williams, B. G., Lloyd-Smith, J. O., Gouws, E., Hankins, C. A., Getz, W. M., Hargrove, J., . . . Auvert, B. (2006). The potential impact of male circumcision on HIV in sub-Saharan Africa. *PLoS Medicine, 3*(7), e262.

6

SAYING NO TO PrEP RESEARCH IN MALAWI

What Constitutes 'Failure' in Offshored HIV Prevention Research?[1]

Kristin Peterson, Morenike Oluwatoyin Folayan, Edward Chigwedere, and Evaristo Nthete

Between 2004 and 2005, the first multisite clinical trial tested whether an existing, marketed antiretroviral drug, tenofovir (tenofovir disoproxil fumarate, or TDF), could prevent HIV transmission. Known as pre-exposure prophylaxis (PrEP), several institutions formed partnerships to carry out the research.[2] Family Health International (referred to as FHI in this article, but renamed FHI360 in 2011), an international social marketing firm, administered the trials. Gilead Sciences, the manufacturer, supplied TDF medication, and the Gates Foundation funded most research sites.[3] The trials were offshored to teaching hospitals and research institutions in Cambodia, Nigeria, Cameroon, Ghana, Thailand, and Malawi. Local HIV-negative sex workers and injection drug users (in Thailand) were recruited as trial volunteers due to their perceived high-risk behavior. Most PrEP trials prematurely shut down for several reasons. Planned and ongoing trials in Cambodia, Cameroon, and Nigeria respectively ended within months of each other (Mills et al., 2005). Thailand and Ghana were the only sites that concluded the trial. Ghana had inconclusive results (L. Peterson et al., 2007) and Thailand showed promising results (Choopanya et al., 2013) although it was hampered by claims of extreme ethical problems (Jintarkanon, Nakapiew, Tienudom, Suwannawong, & Wilson, 2005; Kaplan, 2009). Two of these trial sites caught international attention – Cambodia and Cameroon (Chase, 2005; Chippaux, 2005; Grant et al., 2005; Jintarkanon et al., 2005; Lange, 2005). In Cambodia, a national sex workers' union, the Women's Network for Unity (WNU), made its complaints about the trial protocol clear in national and international press conferences (Forbes & Mudaliar, 2009; Rosengarten & Michael, 2009; Sandy, 2012). The most important issue for WNU was side effects. Given their poor earning status and little access to health care, WNU members argued that any possible illness even over the short term could very quickly create hardship and economic instability for their families (Forbes & Mudaliar, 2009; Sandy, 2012). WNU asked the trial coordinators for 20–30 years of insurance that would cover trial-related illnesses if they were to participate (Forbes & Mudaliar, 2009). While trial coordinators appeared to be sympathetic, the trial protocol was not modified to match these requests (Forbes & Mudaliar, 2009).

In Cameroon, longtime AIDS activists also raised several similar concerns pertaining mostly to the protocol design. These concerns included the fact that protocol and informed consent documents were written only in English and not French (Cameroon's two official languages); female condoms were not included in the protocol; no provisions were made for the care of trial participants if they sero-converted during the trial; and there were no stipulations on future access to drugs if proven effective (Yomgne, 2009). As in Cambodia, activists suggested modifications to the protocol to allay these concerns, which did not materialize. These issues were soon overshadowed by attention brought to the Cameroonian media's misconstrued portrayals of the trials (Mack, Robinson, MacQueen, Moffett, & Johnson, 2010; Yomgne, 2009), which appeared while negotiations were taking place between activists and researchers. Subsequently, the governments of Cambodia and Cameroon shut down the trials. Official reasons for trial closures were not entirely clear in both cases.

Despite the contentious points raised about the research protocol and its design, local actors who raised concerns were consistently portrayed as unable to understand clinical science. Specifically, scientists outside these countries and working within international HIV prevention consortiums insisted that communities required more HIV science education. It was thought that once communities could better understand the principles of HIV clinical research, there would be no unnecessary failure to implement PrEP trials (Grant et al., 2005; Mills et al., 2005; UNAIDS, 2007). Such communities were imagined to be AIDS activists and sex workers.

But in Malawi and Nigeria, the communities that raised similar and more extended questions about these initial PrEP trials were university ethicists and research scientists. The contentions raised in both these countries received relatively little if any attention in the media and the international scientific literature (Chigwedere, 2009; Ukpong, 2009). With this conspicuous absence, our research project endeavored to understand the debates in both these sites. In this article, we focus solely on events that took place in Malawi and analyze why two Malawian ethics committees – one national and constituent of the Ministry of Health, another based at the University of Malawi's College of Medicine – not only denied ethics approval for the planned PrEP study in 2005, but also twice again in 2009.

Our ethnographic and archival work took place between 2005 and 2011. At international AIDS conferences and HIV research meetings, we conducted participant observation and interviewed members of international HIV prevention consortiums as well as feminist activists who first coined the term 'microbicide' – compounds used in the vagina or rectum that were tested for HIV prevention mostly during the 2000s. We interviewed scientists who conducted preclinical PrEP research in the 1990s as well as scientists and ethicists at relevant research institutions – those who designed protocols and those who implemented them at research sites. In Nigeria and Malawi, we interviewed trial workers, state and university ethicists, and trial volunteers. We also followed and analyzed extensive debates on microbicide and PrEP trials taking place on African listservs (see especially the Nigeria HIV Vaccine and Microbicide Advocacy Group [NHVMAG], n.d.). We conducted 62 informal and formal open-ended semi-structured interviews over this period. Both Peterson and Folayan have worked together on HIV clinical research in Nigeria since 2004. Prior to this study, they both had established different professional connections in Malawi, which included colleagues working on ethics committees as well as those working in HIV prevention research. These connections facilitated access to the research site, including introductions to potential interviewees.[4]

In Malawi there was a prolonged debate over the scientific rationales of PrEP, which explicitly did not pertain to 'bioethics' – a term used to analyze the standards of clinical practice. This debate circled around differences of opinion between Malawi-based primary investigators (the PIs) and scientists on the Malawi ethics committees (the ethicists). The PIs claimed that PrEP is a potential biomedical HIV prevention strategy that would have important national ramifications; and, as such, they argued that failing to implement an important and needed trial was a substantial setback for research in Malawi. However, the ethicists claimed that PrEP – as a future HIV prevention technology and not the trial itself – is a problematic contradiction to the country's national HIV treatment policy and could worsen the national HIV problem.

It is argued that debates over PrEP science rationales in the Malawi case are embedded in postcolonial politics that have shaped the structural possibilities of scientific research in the African postcolony. The construct of failure has undergirded the arguments and analyses of offshored PrEP research in Malawi and elsewhere – that a trial failed to be implemented; that a national HIV policy could fail; that African publics failed to understand scientific research; or that international PrEP researchers failed to understand African concerns. However, our ethnographic research pointed to a different analytical scale of failure: it is impossible to delink considerations of PrEP as a future prevention technology to other larger issues that the interviewees identified, such as the national economy, research infrastructure and legacies, and global HIV prevention and treatment politics.

This chapter analyzes these points by first describing Malawi's political and economic histories that created the circumstances for the country to become an offshore destination for HIV clinical research. We then link these contexts to Malawi's history of state research regulation for which expertise and clinical capacities differently evolved to shape debates over scientific rationales. Second, we describe the three multisite PrEP trials that were denied IRB approval in Malawi, while all other sites throughout African and Asian countries gave IRB approval; and we draw on ethnographic fieldwork and interviews to detail the stakes. This article concludes by analyzing the implications of these debates: the concept of failure needs to expand beyond bioethical frames and clinical practices to also include the politics, research visions, structural conditions (Cohen, 1999; Hamdy, 2012), and especially imperial relations that have made HIV research contentions possible.

AIDS intersections: Foreign funding, African economic crisis, and offshore clinical research

Malawi is a southern African country whose colonial and postcolonial history has framed the context of institutionalized medicine and clinical research. Under colonial Nyasaland (now Malawi), those seeking medical training and expertise traveled to medical schools in Northern Rhodesia (now Zambia) and Southern Rhodesia (now Zimbabwe) (Broadhead & Muula, 2002). This education migration created a significant brain drain and, in response, the state of Malawi built a medical school – the College of Medicine at the University of Malawi – in the mid-1980s to ensure student retention and institutionalize scientific research (Broadhead & Muula, 2002). These efforts required foreign funding and participation, which was obtained from British, West German, Australian, Dutch, and Malawian governments (Broadhead & Muula, 2002). These early aid packages mark one of the first iterations of foreign-determined research agendas inside Malawian research institutes. For instance, the curriculum focus was determined by the funders and geared toward community-based medicine, which was welcomed at the time and continues to be the foundation of Malawi's medical education (Broadhead & Muula, 2002).

But by the early 1990s, foreign aid funding priorities began to change, and subsidies for medical institutions were withdrawn (Broadhead & Muula, 2002; Wendland, 2010). These changes in foreign aid were influenced by politics emerging at the end of the Cold War such that Malawi and other Southern African countries were no longer viewed as needing to be coaxed against Soviet influence. Making matters worse, the repressive actions of the Kumuzu Banda regime (1961–1994) neglected the health and research sectors, leading to steady deterioration (Wendland, 2010). Toward the end of his regime, AIDS was hitting Malawi very hard. By 2003, 14% of adults were living with HIV, making Malawi, along with other Southern African countries, the center of the global AIDS epidemic (Craddock, 2000; Kalipeni & Ghosh, 2007; Watkins, 2004). By the mid-1990s the economy worsened even further largely due to the implementation of the International Monetary Fund's structural adjustment program or SAP (Kalipeni, 2004; Wendland, 2010). SAPs installed throughout Africa mandated currency devaluation, the removal of public funds, and privatization of health services, which led to worker retrenchment, massive national debt, and tumultuous household poverty (Mkandawire & Soludo, 1998; K. Peterson, 2014; Turshen, 1999). Malawi's national economy, based primarily on agriculture and a large labor migration into neighboring country mines, grew increasingly stressed. Kalipeni (2004) describes how a radical withdrawal of state funds from the public sector made it extraordinarily difficult for Malawian health and research institutions to be funded and to function (see also Wendland, 2010).

As the AIDS crisis and the impoverishment that came with structural adjustment converged, foreign funding to scattered HIV/AIDS nongovernmental organizations began to be administered. Such funding haphazardly supported the provision of some health-care services that broken health-care systems could no longer address (Benton, 2015; Nguyen, 2010; Smith, 2014). Over time, AIDS interventions were justified via discourses that articulated the urgent and growing humanitarian crisis as a predicament of African governments' inability to manage increasing HIV infections. As Vinh-Kim Nguyen (2009) points out, the establishment and scaling up of massive AIDS intervention programs created a paradigm for which entire populations were standardized and targeted for AIDS interventions. He argues that this "humanitarian assemblage of populations constitutes a global biopolitical laboratory that allows a full range of novel technologies (ranging from highly individualized biomedical interventions to policies to juridical systems) to be 'trialed'" (Nguyen, 2009, p. 213).

Following Nguyen's argument, we concur that PrEP was a significant component of these HIV prevention and intervention logics. As early as 1995, activists, scholars, and policymakers working at the intersections of gender and development advocated for novel biomedical HIV prevention research geared toward protecting and empowering women who were disproportionately affected by the epidemic (Forbes, 2013; Heise & Elias, 1995). The urgency of this gender-based advocacy inadvertently mapped onto the globalization of clinical trials. The tremendous expansion of clinical molecules (made available via technological advances in combinatorial chemistry) were outsourced to the private sector as well as offshored to countries outside of high-earning pharmaceutical markets (Fisher, 2009; Petryna, 2009; Sunder Rajan, 2012). This increased clinical trial activity is directly connected to the brand-name pharmaceutical industry's strategy of expanding pharmaceutical uses and their markets (Dumit, 2012). The strategy to sustain market share includes treating chronic diseases (Dumit, 2012) such as HIV as well as expanding the use of anti-AIDS drugs, which includes PrEP.[5]

In light of these convergences between the dispossession of African research infrastructures, HIV gendered urgencies, and the exponential increase of clinical trials, Malawi became a desirable destination to host trials as well as to draw on a population of volunteers to carry out clinical research. As a funding gap for medical research and training emerged, institutions in the U.S. (and other countries) stepped in to draw on Malawi's existing scientific expertise as well as partner with the country's medical and research facilities. But unlike Malawi's earlier history, the research institutions did not establish agendas that focused on community-based health. In fact, the country does not have an actual strategic plan geared toward research that addresses national health priorities (Kirigia, Kathyola, Muula, & Ota, 2015). Rather, foreign partners established and financed more or less permanent institutions that mostly fund high-priority global health research (Muula & Mfutso-Bengo, 2007). That is, "much of the research on human subjects in Malawi is in the discipline of infectious diseases, mostly tuberculosis, HIV and AIDS, other sexually transmitted infections, and malaria. Research on non-communicable diseases such as diabetes, hypertension and cancer is almost non-existent" (Muula & Mfutso-Bengo, 2007, p. 35).

Two major Malawi-based U.S. institutions are noteworthy because they were involved in the PrEP trials. The first is the University of North Carolina (UNC) Project–Malawi, which has been collaborating with the Ministry of Health since

1990. It is based at the Kamuzu Central Hospital campus in Lilongwe and employs over 250 research scientists and medical personnel (University of North Carolina Project Malawi, n.d.). The second is John Hopkins University's Bloomberg School of Public Health, which partners with the University of Malawi's College of Medicine and the Ministry of Health. This collaboration began in 1988 and focuses primarily on HIV transmission research (Malawi College of Medicine–Johns Hopkins University Research Project, n.d.).[6] It is based in the city of Blantyre and employs over 200 staff members, including researchers, nurses, clinicians, and laboratory personnel (Malawi College of Medicine–Johns Hopkins University Research Project, n.d.).[7]

HIV research projects directed by FHI as well as worldwide consortiums, including the Microbicides Trial Network and the HIV Prevention Trials Network (HPTN), were designed to "evaluate new HIV prevention interventions and strategies in populations and geographical regions that bear a disproportionate burden of infection" (HTPN, n.d.). The Blantyre and Lilongwe research centers have hosted each of these networks' trials in the past. The partnerships interfaced with existing Malawian research regulatory bodies, which became the central locale for debates over PrEP in Malawi.

Offshore research encounters and Malawian national research regulation

Research regulation in Malawi began in 1974, when the National Research Council of Malawi was established by presidential decree (Ndebele & Mfutso-Benga, 2007). The National Commission on Science and Technology (NCST) was also constituted at that time to promote and regulate research in Malawi (NCST, n.d.). Between 1974 and 1994, the NCST reviewed all protocols for research implementation in Malawi. In 1994, the research protocol review was decentralized to the specific ministry of concern (such as agriculture and engineering) with the exception of health research, because of its 'sensitive nature' (Muula & Mfutso-Bengo, 2007). Health research involves the recruitment of human participants and therefore requires more detailed scrutiny and review. The National Health Science Research Committee (NHSRC) was then constituted by the NCST to review research protocols on its behalf (NCST, n.d.). The NCST continued to provide oversight function to NHSRC. In this capacity, according to our interviewees of the ethics committees, it has the power to play the role of an arbitrator when disputes over research protocols arise between the ethics committee and researchers.

In 1991, the University of Malawi, College of Medicine, was established. Initially, research protocols that emanated from this medical school was reviewed by the NHSRC until 1997, when a new institutional review board (IRB) – the College of Medicine Research and Ethics Committee (COMREC) – was established in the medical school (Muula & Mfutso-Bengo, 2007). Two members of COMREC sit on the NHSRC committee, and two members of the NHSRC sit on the COMREC committee (COMREC, n.d.). The membership overlap was established to allow for a functional interaction between the university and national research regulatory organs. These two ethics committees are expected not only to review health-related research protocols, but also to monitor their implementation (COMREC, n.d.).

We were informed by several interviewees that the collaboration between these two IRBs had worked well in the past, but foreign PrEP protocols submissions brought unprecedented confusions and tensions to light. Specifically, COMREC's mandate is to review research proposals that originate from the medical school (Muula & Mfutso-Bengo, 2007). However, this committee refers all clinical studies of 'national interest' and those with political sensitivity to the NHSRC; examples of national interest studies can include vaccine trials, drug trials, stem cell research, genetic studies, and national surveys (Ndebele & Mfutso-Benga, 2007). According to a member of the National Commission for Science and Technology, most research may constitute 'national interest,' but there are additional concerns regarding health and safety. That is, if anything "goes wrong," as he put it, a federal agency that approves a protocol puts responsibility on the government rather than the research institution. If a study is deemed of national interest, then a special committee comprising members of both ethics review boards is set up to review protocols (Ndebele & Mfutso-Benga, 2007).

With the arrival of PrEP, a number of unprecedented disputes emerged that were couched within a seemingly peculiar dichotomy that is elaborated upon below: the enrichment of Malawian national research versus the integrity of HIV national policies. These disputes can be linked to Malawi's political history for which clinical, medical, and research institutions have been tied to foreign funding, which has had two effects. One is that foreign financing has provided sustained funds for research as well as opportunities for increasing international collaborations. Second, there has been a growing development of research and ethics specialists in Malawi whose expertise got institutionalized within medical institutions and state regulation. This expertise arose as a result of longtime experience with community-based medicine and clinical medical practice. But it was especially influenced by the know-how that ethicists developed as a result of the exponential increase in off-shored research protocols (Petryna, 2009) that were showing up in Malawian and other African institutional review boards.[8] The simultaneous development of these two factors meant that while Malawian-based scientists could expertly scrutinize foreign research protocols, state research institutions did not have the capacity to define and implement nationally determined health research priorities. This gap gave rise to unforeseen predicaments in health research – problems that would ultimately stake claims over the question of failure and HIV research.

Tenofovir (TDF) and Truvada PrEP knock on Malawi's door

In 2004 and in 2009, the University of Malawi College of Medicine received three research protocols to study TDF (submitted in 2004 and 2009) and Truvada (submitted in 2009) as PrEP. At that time, both pharmaceuticals were existing marketed nucleoside reverse transcriptase inhibitors used to treat HIV infection. None of these research protocols received IRB approval in Malawi. The same protocols were, however, approved, and the studies were implemented in other African countries. FHI was supposed to conduct the first 2004 study. A second protocol submitted by FHI in 2009 was called FEMPREP, and the planned study drug was Truvada (a combination pill containing the U.S. FDA-approved marketed antiretrovirals, Emtricitabine and TDF).[9] The intention was to assess the safety and effectiveness of the daily use of Truvada in preventing HIV in women who were considered to be at high risk of infection. That same year, the Microbicide Trials Network submitted another protocol, called VOICE,[10] which intended to use Truvada and TDF as study products.[11]

The 2004 TDF trial was to be conducted by the University of North Carolina Project Malawi. It was a phase II PrEP study and was initially granted approval on 7 September 2004 by the University of Malawi's IRB, COMREC. During the initial IRB deliberations, questions were raised about the prospect of drug resistance. After UNC addressed COMREC's concerns on this matter, the protocol was approved. Upon approval, formative research within a nearby community commenced, which generated data on the acceptability of TDF as PrEP among potential recruits. Those who conducted this research informed the authors that they identified sex workers located in 90 different brothels, lounges, and bars that they frequented. The implementation of the phase II study was deemed highly favorable.

Yet, on 24 November 2005, about 14 months after the approval of the protocol and before the trial enrolled participants, the NHSRC chair informed UNC via an official letter that the study's IRB approval had been withdrawn. From the letter, the NHSRC Chair cites "advice received from specialist HIV management groups of the Ministry of Health (MoH) and a presentation on TDF from UNC on 18 November 2005" as reasons for study discontinuation. The withdrawal of ethics approval happened before the recruitment of study participants actually commenced. We were repeatedly told by local PIs that the reasons for withdrawal had to do with 'national interest.' The PIs claimed that there was no other communication beyond this explanation.

Four years later, the FEMPREP and VOICE study protocols were submitted for ethical reviews. Both were submitted to COMREC, which forwarded these applications to NHSRC because they were both deemed to be of 'national interest.' This marked the beginning of what appeared to be several lengthy delays and a great deal of confusion on how the research protocols were handled, including how the ethics committees communicate with the researchers. The ethics committees raised several issues with the FEMPREP and VOICE study protocols. According to our findings from interviews with ethics committee members and researchers, the main concern related to the possibility of promoting HIV resistance to the study drug. A second concern had to do with what are known as 'post-trial benefits.' In this case, these included whether the country of Malawi could easily access the drug if the trial results were successful – an issue not brought up during our interviews but discussed in official IRB documents exchanged between the ethics committees and the PIs. Several open and closed meetings took place over an 18-month period. In the end, the NHSRC refused to give approval for both protocols.

Ultimately, the National Commission for Science and Technology (NCST), which is the overarching national science and research government agency, was asked to arbitrate what was becoming a conflict between the researchers and the national ethics committee. The NCST set up a three-person committee to review the protocols. It also sought external opinions and assessed the situation in other countries that were conducting similar studies. The NCST asserted that concern over resistance to Truvada within the frame of the HIV prevention protocol was not reason enough to stop the implementation of the trials based on the evidence generated from the various reports received. The NCST does not have the authority to override NHSRC decisions; it could only advise the NHSRC to review its decision.

In early 2010, and in a new twist of events, the NHSRC requested that the researchers secure a no-fault health insurance in the case of HIV positive seroconversion and resistance. The intent was to guard against the potential negative impact on study participants' health that could occur well after the PrEP study had been concluded. The NHSRC stated that this requirement is in line with guidance point 19 of the Council for International Organizations of Medical Sciences International Ethical Guidelines. While researchers for the proposed FEMPREP and VOICE studies managed to secure health insurance for study participants, the NHSRC did not grant approval for either of the trials. Ultimately, the main point of contention remained with the question of drug resistance and, to a lesser extent, the question of access to products if deemed successful after being trialed in Malawi. But both drug resistance and post-trial benefits indexed far greater issues shaping research and health outcomes.

The debate: Drug resistance, post-trial benefits, foreign funding

In 2004, when FHI submitted the first TDF protocol for ethics approval, it did not stipulate monitoring drug resistance if trial participants were to seroconvert. But as later PrEP protocols began to include drug-resistance monitoring, researchers were quite reassured by the apparent enhanced safety of these drugs due to the comparably low toxicity and the low levels of drug resistance. Indeed, the researchers in Malawi meant to administer these trials locally echoed to us and in their statements to, and meetings with, COMREC and the NHSRC, that drug resistance was a fairly negligible issue. For example, one senior trial worker explained:

> We did a mathematical modeling on answering that question on resistance. Tenofovir has a very huge barrier for developing resistance. And between Blantyre and Lilongwe we were going to recruit 150 participants on the study drug and another 150 would be on placebo.
>
> Resistance to Tenofovir is much lower than resistance to Combivir and 3TC or D4T and 3TC. So we worked that out of the 150 [trial participants], probably 1 person would develop resistance during the study – 1 out 150. So therefore, there is no way you can say that you unleash a huge resistance burden within Malawi. It's either these participants would be followed rigorously

> during the study and if we saw any resistance we would send samples to our partners to work out which regimen would be the best suited to this participant. [Therefore] we answered those questions.

But the IRBs were not simply concerned about resistance that could arise within an imagined isolated context of a drug trial. They were concerned about the fact that in Malawi, a country that provides universal access to antiretroviral treatment for HIV infection, TDF was part of the second and last line of therapy in the national HIV treatment policy.[12] HIV-positive patients usually begin with one treatment combination, and when HIV becomes resistant to this first line therapy, the patient will switch to a new HIV drug combination, or a second-line treatment. For Malawi, if a trial volunteer was to develop a TDF-resistant HIV strain, no treatment in-country would be available to him or her. Another researcher we interviewed indicated that the research team addressed this concern:

> We had responded to them and told them that the world moves too fast and the treatment of HIV is moving too fast for anybody to think that treatment which is available today may be the same treatment that could be used next year. More efficacious treatment is coming up. Even if Tenofovir was found to be effective we were sure that by the time a good number of Malawians will need Tenofovir as a 2nd line, Tenofovir will not be 2nd line, there would be something more efficacious than Tenofovir so there is nothing to worry about. But people were worried about it.

One IRB member, echoing several ethics committee members' sentiments, explained at length that ultimately the problem was rooted in managing HIV-resistant strains when the drugs needed to do so were not available in Malawi:

> We know that [with] any drug, a person will develop resistance as time goes on – that is a given fact. . . . But it's the mode of resistance development, the source of resistance development that is a worry or reason for concern. This is not a treatment trial, it's a trial on PrEP and this is a low income country. As a low-income country you are using this 2nd line [treatment] drug regimen for PrEP and there is no mechanisms for substitution in the future from the government coffers. You sacrifice a vital drug in the 2nd line regimen, which is expensive. You see, you are caught in a dilemma – you have to promote science and at the same time you are very poor. . . . We needed to address the issue that if we sacrifice this drug these people will have no option, no alternatives if they resist . . . the 1st line. . . . The issue is about sacrificing the best available alternative. . . . To me the issue of resistance is not an issue . . . [because] the resistance argument is becoming weaker and weaker.

At this point one of us asked why the resistance argument is actually weaker. He emphasized again that drug resistance for HIV treatment is an expected outcome that a poor country such as Malawi can certainly anticipate, but for which it cannot develop a treatment policy simply because it does not have the funding to do so. It would require what he called "drug sacrifice." Indeed, national treatment policies in low-income countries such as Malawi are determined not only by advances in new treatments but by their affordability for countrywide HIV treatment programs. In most cases, first line drugs are off-patent, generic, and far less expensive. These drugs destined for large HIV-positive populations can be more easily secured than many of the second-line and most third-line drug treatments (referred to as "salvage therapy"), which are patented and far less affordable. At the time of this study, Malawi had only one second-line option and no salvage therapy regimen recommendation, because such drugs are not affordable.

At least two interviewees mentioned that the national media were discussing the possibility of Malawi losing its next round of United Nations Global Fund financing, the largest funding source for HIV treatment in Malawi. Without such financing, people living with HIV and receiving antiretroviral drugs that are funded by the Global Fund run the risk of having their 'lifelong' treatment terminated. And so the tension between promoting science and good health outcomes while at 'the same time you are very poor' is a significant postcolonial ethical dilemma for which the structure of research and HIV financial flows present no easy solutions.

But while ethics committee members were concerned about the politics of treatment, researchers involved with PrEP repeatedly indicated that it would be a big loss to Malawi if PrEP research was not pursued there – a sentiment not echoed by the members of the ethics committees. Many of the interviewees could not strongly pinpoint reasons for these opinions, but two did stand out. One was that if PrEP use in Malawi was officially approved based on studies conducted outside of Malawi, local evidence would still need to be generated to inform PrEP-related drug policies and program rollouts.[13] Perhaps more important to these researchers was the second reason: the politics of international funding that underlie the long-term buoyancy of research institutions. As one researcher put it:

> It just set HIV backwards. I think we should have been in there with the rest of the world at the forefront of high tech research. [But instead] we lose out on our capacity building, lose out in terms of our health services system. Research in Malawi is also a big employer . . . we have got cadres [at] all levels. We have got nurses, clinicians, we have lab people, we have data people – and all those people lose out. And particularly for the country we lose out in response to what we do in public health problems in a very strong manner.[14]

This researcher echoed what many had articulated to us – that foreign partnerships fundamentally keep skilled labor employed, bolster the integrity of public and population health, and provide an 'equalizing effect' (often via state-encouraged technology transfers – data sharing, publication opportunities, and equipment provisions) between wealthy research institutes and Malawian scientific institutions

(Muula & Mfutso-Bengo, 2007; NCST, n.d.). Thus, there is a lot at stake in 'losing out.'

In a separate manner, 'losing out' was extended to 'post-trial benefits,' which were not included in the IRB documents and were a concern for both ethics committees. Post-trial benefits pertain to memorandum of understandings or other official assurances that PrEP can be easily accessed by the trial community or host country if found effective; and in this particular case, this assurance was relevant only if connected to the non-trial-related issue of securing an alternative to the second-line antiretroviral treatment for trial volunteers who become infected with resistant strains. But offshored PrEP research is rarely connected to post-trial benefits that must engage the politics of global drug marketing where patented drugs are sold on private high-income markets; they are rarely sold on low-income markets and are instead available only via limited free donor programs (K. Peterson, 2014). This disconnect has to do with the fact that drug companies do not play direct roles in PrEP research, but rather they donate their pharmaceutical products to clinical trials. This kind of brokerage places several institutions between the drug company and the study volunteers, making it very difficult to assure access to future drugs and health care (Fisher, 2009; Petryna, 2009; Sunder Rajan, 2007).

Conclusion

During the early PrEP trials and debates, discussions of trial failure have been strongly influenced by the urgency to take global action against HIV (UNAIDS, 2007). PrEP trial failure has been relegated to a problem of activists and the media who do not understand research and who block or disrupt lifesaving research (Chase, 2005; Grant et al., 2005; Mack et al., 2010). Failure is also about trial sponsors and PIs' inability to understand scientific and ethical analysis by communities where trials are offshored (Jintarkanon et al., 2005; Ukpong & Peterson, 2009). Failure pertains to the functions of (bio)ethics, which has been analyzed by scholars (and edited volumes) as variable, singular and universal, context driven, and embedded in regulation, knowledge production, economic disparities, and political economy, to name a few (Cohen, 1999; Cooper & Waldby, 2014; Fisher, 2009; Geissler, 2015; Geissler & Molyneux, 2011; Hamdy, 2012; Kingori, 2013; Molyneux & Geissler, 2008; Petryna, 2009; Sunder Rajan, 2012; Rosengarten & Michael, 2013). Failure might be inevitable (or not), given the inequalities found between wealthy overseas research institutions and their impoverished neighboring communities and research collaborators (Crane, 2013; Fairhead, Leach, & Small, 2006; Farmer, 2002; Geissler, Kelly, Imoukhuede, & Pool, 2008; Gikonyo, Bejon, Marsh, & Molyneux, 2008; Reynolds, Cousins, Newell, & Imrie, 2013; Wendland, 2008).[15]

In analyzing the politics of PrEP in Malawi, we wish to draw upon many of these insights, especially those of Cooper and Waldby (2014), Fisher (2009), and Sunder Rajan (2007; 2012), who examine the politics of neoliberalism and imperialism when it comes to offshored and privatized research. Our analysis does not explicitly pertain to bioethics or ethical variability. As shown, the Malawi debates focused on

PrEP science rationales. These debates were connected primarily to national HIV policies and the ability to secure long-term funding for second-line and salvage therapy; and secondarily, they were connected to the possibility of creating agreeable terms to access marketed drug products that are tested in Malawi. Here, the issues raised did not pertain to trial practices and easily identifiable inequalities. Rather, the question was whether PrEP as a HIV prevention technology (and not a clinical trial) could be reconciled with broader questions of future research agendas, future drugs, and future national health concerns. In taking PrEP debates to this more macro level, the analytical scale of ethics shifts from trial relationships to the postcolonial legacies – geopolitics and economic liberalization – that structure the possibilities of research and health outcomes in Malawi.

How then do we locate 'failure' in this larger field? Genuine desires to develop interventions for HIV prevention must come to terms with the history of Malawi's economic and legal dispossessions and its place in the global economy. That is, failure must be understood within the legacies of imperial power. The debates that pit the enrichment of Malawian national research (and the possibility of 'losing out') against the integrity of HIV national policies (and the possibility of facing 'drug sacrifice') reveal much in this regard. As the discussions demonstrate, some scientists expressed a deep desire to be engaged in 'high tech' research, especially to be at the forefront of cutting-edge HIV solutions. For the ethicists, these shared desires come into conflict with the future prospects of HIV treatment. The sustainability of both scientific research and the national HIV treatment policy is largely dependent upon foreign funding. As such, both HIV research and HIV treatment policy are beholden to foreign research agendas in the absence of a national research policy that defines health research priorities for the country.

These contradictions and rather dramatic constraints at the national level must also be reconciled with the politics of PrEP at a more global level. International scientists and AIDS activists have described PrEP as urgent and lifesaving, especially for marginalized women and sero-discordant couples. This argument converges quite effortlessly with drug development models that increase market share. These models invent new uses of existing marketed products that can extend a drug patent's life. Hence, the Malawi ethics committees' concern over post-trial access to successful drug products must be understood within the broader context of who becomes experimental subjects and who becomes contract labor for products destined for high-earning markets located outside of Africa (Cooper & Waldby, 2014; Sunder Rajan, 2007).

Here we might wonder what it means for a Malawian ethics committee to say no to PrEP research, not once but three times. This is not simply about a failure to listen or understand what is at stake in refusing to approve PrEP study protocols. It is about the way in which imperialist relations are constituted via disparate articulations of scientific expertise and civil society, foreign influence, and the African nation-state (which has not 'failed,' as it has made strong claims in the PrEP debates). While there are differently located subjectivities emerging out of this field of power, all actors discursively and materially vie to establish authority over sovereign notions of public health and ultimately the public good. In this context, saying no to PrEP research means understanding the structures of power that make clinical encounters appear completely natural; and as such, they get understood as humanitarian/scientific urgencies rather than about imperial relations.

It is noteworthy that none of our interlocutors used the term 'failure' to describe their perspective on events. But as the early literature on the PrEP trials show, the idea of failure is in constant juxtaposition with assumed normative functions – such as how a trial could successfully work or how bioethics should consider performing within multiple contexts and constraints (International AIDS Society, 2005; UNAIDS, 2007). For those who have expectations that offshored research can locate itself in some imagined normative sense of things, failure to implement a trial is sudden, shocking, and out of the normal range of experience. But if refusals are located within imperialism itself, then saying no to PrEP research is anything but failure. It is about attempts to assert some kind of national integrity – an integrity that ultimately is difficult to achieve because a choice must be made between holding on to opportunities for innovative research or defending the integrity of an HIV treatment policy. These are choices and not synergistic givens. Even as choices they are highly limited, because it is not researchers in Malawi who autonomously determine research agendas, nor is it HIV experts who have the power to establish an ideal national HIV treatment policy for a country hit hard by AIDS. These challenges and structural constraints make the lament over 'drug sacrifice' and 'losing out' within long histories of dispossessions and imperial relations all the more salient.

Editor commentary

Kristin Peterson and colleagues turn our attention to the ethics of public health practice, specifically of offshored clinical trials. In this chapter the authors' highlight the following:

- A tension exists between promoting science and good health outcomes, particularly in low-resource economies.
- Research, public health, and health service finances and agendas remain largely determined by international agents (e.g., funders, academic institutions, institutions of global health), a dynamic that has roots in colonial imperialism.
- Foreign partnerships can prove beneficial, as they can keep skilled local labor employed, bolster the integrity of public and population health, and provide an 'equalizing effect' between wealthy international research institutions and less well-resourced local institutions of science and health.
- Resistance to international agendas is often relegated to a "problem of activists and the media," individuals and entities who are considered as trying to block "lifesaving" advancements because they do not to understand science and research.
- Resistance or refusals to internationally run clinical trials (and public health efforts more generally) can be considered as an attempt to assert national integrity.

Notes

1 Reprint of: Kristin Peterson, Morenike Oluwatoyin Folayan, Edward Chigwedere & Evaristo Nthete (2015): Saying 'No' to PrEP research in Malawi: what constitutes 'failure' in offshored HIV prevention research?, Anthropology & Medicine, DOI: 10.1080/13648470.2015.1081377, www.tandfonline.com.

2 These included The Centers for Disease Control and Prevention, the National Institutes of Health, and University of California San Francisco, among others.

3 The Gates Foundation provided $6.5 million for sites in Cameroon, Nigeria, Ghana, Malawi and Cambodia. The National Institutes of Health awarded $2.1 million to UC San Francisco to conduct a trial in Cambodia. The Center for Disease Control was awarded $3.5 million to conduct the trial in Botswana, Thailand, and the US.

4 National Science Foundation funding enabled Peterson to hire her former colleague, Chigwedere, who brought Nthete on board (both at the University of Malawi, College of Medicine/College of Health Sciences). They were instrumental in identifying interviewees and the research strategy. Together we all contributed to conducting interviews, sharing data, generating analysis, and writing this article. Peterson, Folayan, and Chigwedere travelled to international conferences to conduct research. Peterson, Folayan, and Olatubosun Obileye carried out the research in Nigeria. Chigwedere, Nthete, Folayan, Peterson, and Matilda Kunthi carried out research in Malawi. Peterson and Folayan and analyzed the majority of the data. Both the research and the publication received ethical approval from the University of California, Irvine, US; Obafemi Awolowo University in Ile-Ife, Nigeria; and the National Health Sciences Research Council in Lilongwe, Malawi.

5 The drug industry has been intricately tied to the investment industry since the 1980s, which has demanded short-term gains and high rates of appreciation in return for finance capital. These are demands that are relatively difficult to meet given the risks and long-term need to bring a drug to market (10-15 years). Drug companies survive these demands by merging and acquiring others. It also seeks ways to develop blockbuster drugs - those earning over $1 billion per year (on all these points, see Cooper, 2008; Dumit, 2012; K. Peterson, 2014; Sunder Rajan, 2012).

6 In addition to HIV prevention research, these institutes conduct a wide range of studies including breast feeding, HIV resistance studies, lymphoma, Kaposi's Sarcoma, mother-to-child HIV transmission, vaccine trials, and microbicide use (Malawi College of Medicine–Johns Hopkins University Research Project, n.d.).

7 For other examples of semi-permanent and permanent foreign research institutions in Africa, see Fairhead, Leach, and Small (2006) and Reynolds et al. (2013).

8 While we do not have statistics, one ethicist in Malawi and two in Nigeria noted the substantial increase in the number of foreign research protocols seeking permission to conduct clinical trials from the early 2000s.

9 FEMPREP was a multi-center, double-blind, randomized, placebo-controlled effectiveness and safety study. The trial "assigned 2120 HIV-negative women in Kenya, South Africa, and Tanzania to receive either a combination of tenofovir disoproxil fumarate and emtricitabine (TDF-FTC) or placebo once daily. The primary objective was to assess the effectiveness of TDF-FTC in preventing HIV acquisition and to evaluate safety" (Van Damme et al., 2012, p. 411).

10 VOICE was a Phase 2B, five-arm, double-blinded, placebo-controlled, multi-site, randomized, controlled trial. The trial "assess(ed) daily treatment with oral tenofovir disoproxil fumarate (TDF), oral tenofovir-emtricitabine (TDF-FTC), or 1% tenofovir (TFV) vaginal gel as pre-exposure prophylaxis against HIV-1 infection in women in South Africa, Uganda, and Zimbabwe" (Marrazzo et al., 2015).

11 At both the Johns Hopkins Blantyre site and the UNC Lilongwe site, these included HTPN 035 (a Vaginal Microbicides gel, which began enrollment in 2005 and concluded in 2008), MTN 015 (a Study of Women following HIV-1 Seroconversion in Microbicide Trials), MTN 019 (a study of Tenofovir gel in pregnancy, which is currently pending approval). Currently at the UNC Lilongwe site, the trial MTN 020 is testing a vaginal ring that contains the non-nucleoside reverse transcriptase inhibitor, Dapivirine. The Network had conducted a microbicide trial in Malawi in the past using non-antiretorviral based compounds called buffergel and PRO2000.

12 At the time, the HIV treatment policy's first line standard regimen is a Stavudine (d4T) C Lamivudine (3TC) C Nevirapine (NVP) dose. It also lists three alternatives. The second line (for adults) includes Zidovudine (AZT) C Lamivudine (3TC) C Tenofovir (TDF) C Lopinavir/ Ritonavir (LPV/r). At least up until 2008, there were no alternative formulations to the second line, nor was a third-line regimen established. See Ministry of Health, Malawi (2008).

13 For example, a Niverapine – an antiretroviral used to prevent mother-to-child HIV transmission – study (Eshleman et al., 2005) in Malawi showed that there was high resistance after a single dose of therapy in contrast to other African countries where there was little or significantly less resistance.

14 See Folayan and Allman (2011) on industrial labor in clinical trials.

15 For colonial institutional relations, see Feierman & Janzen, 1992; Hunt, Appadurai, Comaroff, & Farquhar, 1999; Packard, 1989; and Vaughan, 1991.

References

Benton, A. (2015). *AIDS Exceptionalism: Development through Disease in Sierra Leone.* Minneapolis: University of Minnesota Press.

Broadhead, R. L., & Muula, A. S. (2002). Creating a medical school for Malawi: problems and achievements. *BMJ, 325*(7360), 384–387. doi:10.1136/bmj.325.7360.384

Chase, M. (2005). Tenofovir Prevention Study Problems: AIDS Scientists, Activists Fail to Fully Resolve Rift Over Trials. *Wall Street Journal, May 24.*

Chigwedere, E. (2009). The Malawi story. In M. Ukpong & K. Peterson (Eds.), *Oral Tenofovir Controversy II.* Lagos: NVHMAS.

Chippaux, J.-P. (2005). Pharmaceutical Colonialism in Africa. *Le Monde Diplomatique, August.*

Choopanya, K., Martin, M., Suntharasamai, P., Sangkum, U., Mock, P.A., Leethochawalit, M., ... Vanichseni, S. (2013). Antiretroviral prophylaxis for HIV infection in injecting drug users in Bangkok, Thailand (the Bangkok Tenofovir Study): A randomised, double-blind, placebo-controlled phase 3 trial. *Lancet, 381*(9883), 2083–2090. doi:10.1016/s0140-6736(13)61127-7

Cohen, L. (1999). Where it hurts: Indian material for an ethics of organ transplantation. *Daedalus, 128*(4), 135–165.

COMREC (College of Medicine Research and Ethics Committee, University of Malawi). (n.d.). *The Relationship between CoMREC's* (sic) *and NHSRC.* Retrieved from http://www.medcol.mw/comrec/the-relationship-between-comrecs-and-nhsrc-2/

Cooper, M. (2008). *Life as Surplus: Biotechnology and Capitalism in the Neoliberal Era.* Seattle: University of Washington Press.

Cooper, M., & Waldby, C. (2014). *Clinical Labor: Tissue Donors and Research Subjects in the Global Bioeconomy.* Durham, NC: Duke University Press.

Craddock, S. (2000). Disease, social identity, and risk: Rethinking the geography of AIDS. *Transactions of the Institute of British Geographers, 25*(2), 153–168. doi:10.1111/j.0020-2754.2000.00153.x

Crane, J. (2013). *Scrambling for Africa: AIDS, Expertise, and the Rise of American Global Health Science*. Ithaca, NY: Cornell University Press.

Dumit, J. (2012). Prescription maximization and the accumulation of surplus health in the pharmaceutical industry: The 'Biomarx' experiment. In K. Sunder Rajan (Ed.), *Lively Capital: Biotechnologies, Ethics and Governance in Global Markets* (pp. 45–92). Durham, NC: Duke University Press.

Eshleman, S. H., Hoover, D. R., Chen, S., Hudelson, S. E., Guay, L. A., Mwatha, A., . . . Taha, T. (2005). Resistance after single-dose nevirapine prophylaxis emerges in a high proportion of Malawian newborns. *AIDS, 19*(18), 2167–2169.

Fairhead, J., Leach, M., & Small, M. (2006). Where techno-science meets poverty: Medical research and the economy of blood in The Gambia, West Africa. *Social Science & Medicine, 63*(4), 1109–1120. doi:10.1016/j.socscimed.2006.02.018

Farmer, P. (2002). Can transnational research be ethical in the developing world? *Lancet, 360*(9342), 1266. doi:10.1016/s0140-6736(02)11357-2

Feierman, S., & Janzen, J. (1992). *The Social Basis of Health and Healing in Africa*. Berkeley: University of California Press.

Fisher, J. (2009). *Medical Research for Hire: The Political Economy of Pharmaceutical Clinical Trials*. New Brunswick, NJ: Rutgers University Press.

Folayan, M. O., & Allman, D. (2011). Clinical trials as an industry and an employer of labour. *Journal of Cultural Economy, 4*(1), 97–104. doi:10.1080/17530350.2011.535376

Forbes, A. (2013). Mobilizing women at the grassroots to shape health policy: A case study of the Global Campaign for Microbicides. *Reproductive Health Matters, 21*(42), 174–183. doi:10.1016/s0968-8080(13)42735-0

Forbes, A., & Mudaliar, S. (2009). Preventing Prevention Trial Failures: A Case Study and Lessons for Future Trials from the 2004 Tenofovir Trial in Cambodia. Retrieved from http://www.global-campaign.org/clientfiles/Cambodia.pdf

Geissler, P. W. (Ed.). (2015). *Para-States and Medical Science: Making African Global Health*. Durham, NC: Duke University Press.

Geissler, P. W., Kelly, A., Imoukhuede, B., & Pool, R. (2008). 'He is now like a brother, I can even give him some blood' – relational ethics and material exchanges in a malaria vaccine 'trial community' in The Gambia. *Social Science & Medicine, 67*(5), 696–707. doi:10.1016/j.socscimed.2008.02.004

Geissler, P. W., & Molyneux, C. (2011). *Evidence, Ethos and Experiment: The Anthropology and History of Medical Research in Africa*. New York: Berghahn Books.

Gikonyo, C., Bejon, P., Marsh, V., & Molyneux, S. (2008). Taking social relationships seriously: Lessons learned from the informed consent practices of a vaccine trial on the Kenyan Coast. *Social Science & Medicine, 67*(5), 708–720. doi:10.1016/j.socscimed.2008.02.003

Grant, R. M., Buchbinder, S., Cates, W., Jr., Clarke, E., Coates, T., Cohen, M. S., . . . Wainberg, M. A. (2005). AIDS. Promote HIV chemoprophylaxis research, don't prevent it. *Science, 309*(5744), 2170–2171. doi:10.1126/science.1116204

Hamdy, S. (2012). *Our Bodies Belong to God: Organ Transplants, Islam, and the Struggle for Human Dignity in Egypt*. Berkeley, CA: University of California Press.

Heise, L. L., & Elias, C. (1995). Transforming AIDS prevention to meet women's needs: A focus on developing countries. *Social Science & Medicine, 40*(7), 931–943.

HTPN (HIV Prevention Trials Network). (n.d.). About the HTPN. Retrieved from http://www.hptn.org/AboutHPTN.htm

Hunt, N. R., Appadurai, A., Comaroff, J. L., & Farquhar, J. (1999). *A Colonial Lexicon*. Durham, NC: Duke University Press.

International AIDS Society. (2005). Building Collaboration to Advance HIV Prevention – Global Consultation on Tenofovir Pre-Exposure Prophylaxis Research: Report of a consultation convened by the International AIDS Society on Behalf of the Bill and Melinda Gates Foundation. Atlanta, GA: US National Institutes of Health and US Centers for Disease Control.

Jintarkanon, S., Nakapiew, S., Tienudom, N., Suwannawong, P., & Wilson, D. (2005). Unethical clinical trials in Thailand: A community response. *The Lancet, 365*(9471), 1617–1618. doi:10.1016/S0140-6736(05)66501-4

Kalipeni, E. (2004). Structural adjustment and the health-care crisis in Malawi. *Proteus: A Journal of Ideas, 21*(1), 23–30.

Kalipeni, E., & Ghosh, J. (2007). Concern and practice among men about HIV/AIDS in low socioeconomic income areas of Lilongwe, Malawi. *Social Science & Medicine, 64*(5), 1116–1127. doi:10.1016/j.socscimed.2006.10.013

Kaplan, K. (2009). The Thailand story. In M. Ukpong & K. Peterson (Eds.), *Oral Tenofovir Controversy II*. Lagos: NVHMAS.

Kingori, P. (2013). Experiencing everyday ethics in context: Frontline data collectors perspectives and practices of bioethics. *Social Science & Medicine, 98*, 361–370. doi:10.1016/j.socscimed.2013.10.013

Kirigia, J. M., Kathyola, D. D., Muula, A. S., & Ota, M. M. (2015). National health research system in Malawi: Dead, moribund, tepid or flourishing? *BMC Health Serv Res, 15*, 126. doi:10.1186/s12913-015-0796-1

Lange, J. M. (2005). We must not let protestors derail trials of pre-exposure prophylaxis for HIV. *PLoS Medicine, 2*(9), e248. doi:10.1371/journal.pmed.0020248

Mack, N., Robinson, E. T., MacQueen, K. M., Moffett, J., & Johnson, L. M. (2010). The exploitation of "Exploitation" in the tenofovir PrEP trial in Cameroon: Lessons learned from media coverage of an HIV prevention trial. *Journal of Empirical Research on Human Research Ethics, 5*(2), 3–19. doi:10.1525/jer.2010.5.2.3

Malawi College of Medicine–Johns Hopkins University Research Project. (n.d.). Retrieved from http://www.jhsph.edu/research/affiliated-programs/malawi-college-of-medicine-johns-hopkins-research-project/

Marrazzo, J., Ramjee, G., Richardson, B., Gomez, K., Mgodi, N., Nair, G., . . . Chirenje, Z. (2015). Tenofovir-based preexposure prophylaxis for HIV infection among African women. *N Engl J Med, 372*(6), 509–518. doi:10.1056/NEJMoa1402269

Mills, E. J., Singh, S., Singh, J. A., Orbinski, J. J., Warren, M., & Upshur, R. E. (2005). Designing research in vulnerable populations: Lessons from HIV prevention trials that stopped early. *British Medical Journal, 331*(7529), 1403–1406. doi:10.1136/bmj.331.7529.1403

Ministry of Health, Malawi. (2008). *Treatment of AIDS: Guidelines for the Use of Antiretroviral Therapy in Malawi*. 3rd ed. Retrieved from http://www.aidstarone.com/sites/default/files/treatment_documents/hiv_treatment_guidelines_malawi_2008.pdf

Mkandawire, T., & Soludo, C. (1998). *Our Continent, Our Future: African Perspectives on Structural Adjustment*. Dakar: Council for the Development of Social Science Research in Africa (CODESRIA).

Molyneux, S., & Geissler, P. W. (2008). Ethics and the ethnography of medical research in Africa. *Soc Sci Med, 67*(5), 685–695. doi:10.1016/j.socscimed.2008.02.023

Muula, A. S., & Mfutso-Bengo, J. M. (2007). Responsibilities and obligations of using human research specimens transported across national boundaries. *J Med Ethics, 33*(1), 35–38. doi:10.1136/jme.2005.012492

NCST (National Commission for Science and Technology). (n.d.). Welcome to NCST. Retrieved from http://www.ncst.mw/welcome-to-ncst/

Ndebele, P., & Mfutso-Benga, J. (2007). Conducting medical research in Malawi: What researchers need to know. In T. Mduluza (Ed.), *A Gateway to Biomedical Research in Africa* (pp. 91–100). New York: Nova Biomedical Books.

Nguyen, V. K. (2009). Government-by-exception: Enrolment and experimentality in mass HIV treatment programmes in Africa. *Social Theory & Health*, 7(3), 196–217. doi:10.1057/sth.2009.12

Nguyen, V. K. (2010). *The Republic of Therapy: Triage and Sovereignty in West Africa's Time of AIDS*. Durham, NC: Duke University Press.

NHVMAG (Nigeria HIV Vaccine and Microbicide Advocacy Group). (n.d.). Phase 2 Trial of Oral Tenofovir Use as a Chemoprophylaxis for HIV Infection in Nigeria: Report of the Outcome of Dialogue Between the Community and Researchers. Retrieved from http://www.nhvmas-ng.org/publication/tdf.pdf

Packard, R. (1989). *White Plague, Black Labor: Tuberculosis and the Political Economy of Health and Disease in South Africa*. Berkeley: University of California Press.

Peterson, K. (2014). *Speculative Markets*. Durham, NC: Duke University Press.

Peterson, L., Taylor, D., Roddy, R., Belai, G., Phillips, P., Nanda, K., . . . Cates, W. (2007). Tenofovir disoproxil fumarate for prevention of HIV infection in women: A phase 2, double-blind, randomized, placebo-controlled trial. *PLoS Clinical Trials*, *2*(5), e27. doi:10.1371/journal.pctr.0020027

Petryna, A. (2009). *When Experiments Travel: Clinical Trials and the Global Search for Human Subjects*. Princeton: Princeton University Press.

Reynolds, L., Cousins, T., Newell, M. L., & Imrie, J. (2013). The social dynamics of consent and refusal in HIV surveillance in rural South Africa. *Social Science & Medicine*, *77*, 118–125. doi:10.1016/j.socscimed.2012.11.015

Rosengarten, M., & Michael, M. (2009). Rethinking the bioethical enactment of medically drugged bodies: Paradoxes of using anti-HIV drug therapy as a technology for prevention. *Science as Culture*, *18*(2), 183–199. doi:10.1080/09505430902885565

Rosengarten, M., & Michael, M. (2013). *Innovation and Biomedicine Ethics, Evidence and Expectation in HIV*. Basingstoke, Hampshire: Palgrave Macmillan.

Sandy, L. (2012). International agendas and sex worker rights in Cambodia. In M. Ford (Ed.), *Social Activism in South East Asia* (pp. 154–169). London: Routledge.

Smith, D. (2014). *AIDS Doesn't Show Its Face: Inequality, Morality, and Social Change in Nigeria*. Chicago: University of Chicago Press.

Sunder Rajan, K. (2007). Experimental values: Indian clinical trials and surplus health. *New Left Review*, *45*(May/June), 67–88.

Sunder Rajan, K. (2012). Pharmaceutical crises and questions of value: Terrains and logics of global therapeutic politics. *South Atlantic Quarterly*, *111*(2), 321–346.

Turshen, M. (1999). *Privatizing Health Services in Africa*. New Brunswick, NJ: Rutgers University Press.

Ukpong, M. (2009). The Nigeria story. In M. Ukpong & K. Peterson (Eds.), *Oral Tenofovir Controversy II: Voices from the Field*. Lagos: NHVMAS.

Ukpong, M., & Peterson, K. (Eds.). (2009). *Oral Tenofovir Controversy II: Voices from the Field*. Lagos: NHVMAS.

UNAIDS. (2007). *Good Participatory Practice Guidelines for Biomedical HIV Prevention Trials*. Geneva: UNAIDS.

University of North Carolina Project Malawi. (n.d.). http://www.med.unc.edu/infdis/malawi.

Van Damme, L., Corneli, A., Ahmed, K., Agot, K., Lombaard, J., Kapiga, S., . . . Taylor, D. (2012). Preexposure prophylaxis for HIV infection among African women. *New England Journal of Medicine*, *367*(5), 411–422. doi:10.1056/NEJMoa1202614

Vaughan, M. (1991). *Curing Their Ills: Colonial Power and African Influence*. Stanford: Stanford University Press.

Watkins, S. C. (2004). Navigating the AIDS epidemic in rural Malawi. *Population and Development Review, 30*(4), 673–705. doi:10.1111/j.1728-4457.2004.00037.x
Wendland, C. L. (2008). Research, therapy, and bioethical hegemony: The controversy over perinatal AZT trials in Africa. *African Studies Review, 51*(3), 1–23. doi:10.1353/arw.0.0084
Wendland, C. L. (2010). *A Heart for the Work: Journeys through an African Medical School.* Chicago: University of Chicago Press.
Yomgne, C.T. (2009). The Cameroon story. In M. Ukpong & K. Peterson (Eds.), *Oral Tenofovir Controversy II.* Lagos: NVHMAS.

7

ORAL HEALTH AS A CITIZEN-MAKING PROJECT

Immigrant Parents' Contestations of Dental Public Health Campaigns

Sarah Horton and Judith Barker

The school nurse called in six of the school's "hard-luck cases" from their classes and had them open their mouths for my benefit. Mrs. Madrigal's child had what the nurse called "the worst teeth in ____ Elementary School." Roberto,[1] now six years old, had been born in Mexico and had arrived in Mendota, California, at the age of one. When he entered kindergarten, he received a dental and physical screening by a county mobile van. The county dentist had marked Roberto's teeth a "1," meaning he required "very urgent treatment" due to oral disease that could cause permanent physical or developmental effects. The school nurse kept a list of these cases and sent a note home to Roberto's mother. That was the beginning of a long history of headaches for both the school nurses and Mrs. Madrigal, mutual frustration caused by a confluence of factors that had all contributed to poor dental hygiene and a lack of eligibility for care.

By the time I met Roberto, he was on his second round of antibiotics to treat the infection in his gums – an anodyne to salve his lack of dental treatment and prevent a systemic infection. His front teeth had rotted to become flush with his gumline. He had two permanent molars scooped out with oral disease and one canine tooth verging on black. He didn't like to smile for his school photograph and had difficulty pronouncing certain words. He had been found to be "slow in language acquisition" and was made to repeat kindergarten.

Mrs. Madrigal recalled the relationship she'd developed with the many officials assigned to her case over the year, summing it up with a nervous laugh and the phrase: "They call me all the time." She received notes from the school and county nurse about Roberto's teeth and phone calls from the social worker with the school district's migrant program. Sometimes, Roberto's teeth began to hurt when he ate his lunch, and a trip to the school nurse would trigger a call to Mrs. Madrigal again. But mostly, said Roberto, a shy child with a sheepish grin, he just ate quietly because he knew that – as he put it – "they can't treat me."

When Roberto first entered school, Mrs. Madrigal had a brief glimmer of hope he might be treated. The county Migrant Program had a small amount of funds to pay for dental treatment, so it covered Roberto's examination by a local dental specialist. At the time of Roberto's visit in November 2003, his chart revealed that he would require "three therapeutic pulpotomies; five prefabricated stainless steel crowns on primary teeth; two two-surface amalgam crowns; one resin filling on two surfaces; one extraction of an erupted tooth; and one space maintainer." Yet, as noted by the specialist, the biggest obstacle to Roberto's treatment was his "lack of cooperation." Treatment objectives were determined based on "visual exam[s]; we couldn't even get him to keep his mouth open for the X-rays." The most expensive aspect of Roberto's care would have been the general anesthesia necessary to perform such extensive treatment on such a young uncooperative child – an $8,000 price tag that the county program could not afford. As a result, Roberto went home without treatment, and the school nurse and the Migrant Program continued sending notes home to Mrs. Madrigal.

By the end of Roberto's first year in kindergarten, school officials were threatening legal action. The school nurse had talked to the migrant program's parent liaison, who had intimated that a Child Protective Services worker could be assigned to Mrs. Madrigal's case. Mrs. Madrigal again made Roberto an appointment with the local dentist, but he was able to do only a cleaning. She would take Roberto to another two dentists in the area within the year. By the winter, she had grown desperate. She took him to a fifth dentist; this man was unable to do more than a general exam. Speaking to me in English, the dentist called Roberto a "clear referral case;" he'd need a specialist because "his mouth is totally bombed out." Exiting the clinic, Mrs. Madrigal said she felt she had hit a brick wall: "Now he's going to go back to school [after break] and we won't have anything to show for all this. It's going to call attention to me again."

Trapped between Roberto's lack of MediCal, California's public health insurance program, and her family's lack of income, Mrs. Madrigal served as a lightning rod for the pent-up frustration of the school nurse and Migrant Program liaison. The school nurse confided to me about farm-working families such as Mrs. Madrigal's: "Though I have to say that I don't really understand that thing about not having the money. Because when you have five families sharing a house and sharing the rent, then how can you not have the money to pay for dental care? I think what they mean by that is that it's just not a priority." Similarly, the county migrant nurse, who had followed Roberto's case for three years, blamed Mrs. Madrigal for not having successfully disciplined Roberto to make him behave during dental visits. She snapped: "One thing you might ask Mrs. Madrigal is whether oral health is a priority for her. You might ask her, 'what do you expect out of your child's health? Do you expect that it can be made better?' The kids are so young, so it's really up to the parents to make them comply."

This case serves as an example of the arguments we present in this chapter regarding the positioning of immigrants in the U.S. public health system. The complex chain of structural obstacles to Roberto's treatment had disappeared in the revelatory judgment of Mrs. Madrigal as, to draw on a term coined by Charles Briggs and Clara Mantini-Briggs, an "unsanitary subject" (2003). The concept refers to the portrayal of individuals who are unwilling (or unable) to adopt modern hygienic practices as unworthy of citizenship. As public health officials deduced Mrs. Madrigal's improper caregiving based on Roberto's poor oral health, Mrs. Madrigal was held responsible for Roberto's inability to obtain dental treatment. In short, not only children's oral disease but also their behavioral issues are chalked up to the immigrant farmworker parents' improper caregiving.

Drawing upon ethnography in a predominantly immigrant community in California, this chapter explores the ways that oral health professionals and educators present compliance with regimens of oral hygiene as a sign of "proper family governance" that indicates their capacity for citizenship. In doing so, however, they ignore the political and economic circumstances that contribute to children's poor oral health. In the case of Roberto, his initial lack of exposure to fluoridated drinking water in Mexico coupled with his current lack of insurance and his family's lack of income ultimately prevented the Madrigals from meeting norms of "sanitary citizenship." While, in the eyes of health officials, Roberto's severe oral disease attested to Mrs. Madrigal's low rating on a hygienic scale of "civilized conduct" (Ong, 1996, p. 738), the Madrigals' lack of insurance and income precluded their ability to have Roberto's teeth restored.

We suggest that public health campaigns' anxieties about immigrant mothers' caregiving practices serve as a potent site for racialized constructions of Mexicans during this second major wave of immigration to the U.S. Because it is viewed as easily preventable, oral disease is a fruitful site in which to examine concerns about immigrants' mothering as illustrative of broader racial anxieties. The reduction of oral disease in developed nations is viewed as one of the major public health triumphs of the past century due to the fluoridation of public water systems and the promotion of preventive oral hygiene practices (USDHHS [U.S. Department of Health and Human Services], 2000). Yet in the U.S., children from minority groups, Latinos in particular, have not benefited as much as other children from these scientific advances. What specific public anxieties do contemporary concerns about immigrant children's oral hygiene speak to, and to what racialization projects do they contribute? Moreover, how do parents variously interpret, accept, or resist health educators' efforts?

Central Valley: A racialized space internal to the nation

To examine how oral hygiene campaigns construct Mexican immigrant families' "deservingness" of citizenship, I, Sarah Horton, conducted interviews and participant-observation with a range of actors involved in farmworker children's oral health. I lived in Mendota, a predominantly immigrant farm-working community in California's Central Valley, between 2005 and 2006. I interviewed public health officials, public health and social service professionals, educators, civic leaders, and immigrant caregivers about their concerns about Latino children's oral hygiene.

In order to fully capture the experiences of immigrant parents and children in the public health and welfare systems as they shuttled in between dentists, school nurses, and Migrant Program liaisons, I also interviewed the parents of five children whom elementary school nurses deemed to be "problem children" due to their persistent and untreated oral disease. Moreover, to gather firsthand data on their interactions, I accompanied parents and children to dental appointments while providing transportation.

Examination of the role of public health officials in crafting discourses about immigrants' proper place in the polity is best complemented by an analysis of such discourses' practical effects. To understand immigrant mothers' interpretations of and responses to the discourses of these citizen-making agencies, I conducted multiple interviews with 26 Mexican immigrant mothers about their interactions with the health-care and welfare bureaucracies in the area. Mothers were randomly selected from a list of addresses and names from a partner study on farmworker occupational health; they were eligible for inclusion in the study if they self-identified as Latina and had a child of five years old or under. I met with each mother at least twice, and conducted successive interviews with selected families. Mothers, who were primarily undocumented, had been in the U.S. an average of nine years; meanwhile their children varied in citizenship status. Together with observations of the interactions between immigrant mothers and public health officials, interviews with such actors created a complex portrait of the way oral hygiene has become a new site for the elaboration of racial distinctions.

Dubbed the "Cantaloupe Capital of the World," Mendota is a predominantly agricultural town in the heart of the fertile San Joaquin or Central Valley, which provides the nation with one-quarter of all its food (Gonzales & McChesney, 2002). However, agricultural communities in California's Central Valley comprise part of an "other California," one far removed from the state's general economic prosperity. While California's agribusiness industry grosses $27 billion a year (Gonzales & McChesney, 2002), the average household income of a farm-working family is less than $19,999 a year (Aguirre International, 2005). Agribusiness companies typically do not offer farmworkers employment benefits such as child care, pension plans, or health care. Thus, to supplement their meager incomes, eligible farmworkers depend upon public agencies providing food coupons, food stamps, preschool, medical care, and unemployment insurance. Because farm-working families are so dependent upon the state to survive, the state ironically wields considerable influence in the daily conduct of undocumented immigrants and their families. Public health and social service agencies thus play a major role in shaping the sense of civic membership of immigrants in farm-working communities and in incorporating them into the nation as "new Americans."

Given their racial segregation and reliance upon the labor of undocumented immigrants, Latino farm-working communities in the Central Valley constitute a symbolically laden internal borderland of sorts. The town of Mendota is 97% Latino (U.S. Census 2010), primarily of Mexican and Central American origins. Like other Central Valley towns, Mendota has long been a destination point for immigrants who have migrated from central Mexico since at least the late 19th century. Yet the federal Bracero Program, which imported 4.6 million agricultural laborers to work in U.S. agriculture between 1942 and 1964, more tightly linked migration networks in the classic sending areas in Mexico to the region (Ngai, 2004). This small town is now a first destination point for many new arrivals, many of them undocumented. Thus health professionals and social service workers commonly speak of Mendota as a liminal space between Mexico and the U.S. – an internal borderland of sorts. While some call it a "migrant labor camp," others refer to it as a "port of entry" for Mexican immigrants.

To control the flow of disease, goods, and bodies through this internal borderland, public health officials and educators in the Central Valley employ public health policing measures in the form of health screenings and quarantines. As Natalia Molina has shown for the selective enforcement of sanitary codes in Los Angeles' Chinatown in the early 20th century, parents in largely migrant areas are held to a higher standard of healthiness than those in other California communities (2006, pp. 17–45). For example, the state mandates childhood vaccinations. However, proof of a negative tuberculosis (TB) test upon entering kindergarten varies from county to county. Counties with high immigrant populations such as Fresno County require proof of a negative TB test before a child may enter kindergarten. In the Mendota Unified School District, however, school officials have adopted stricter policies, requiring a negative TB test each year before enrollment. In addition, teachers are requested to notify the School Nurse of all children who are leaving the country – mostly to visit Mexico – and the child must be retested after each trip before being readmitted to school. The school district also holds medical and dental screenings for its migrant children at the beginning of the school year, and schools often deny entry to or exclude children with health conditions deemed persistent or contagious, including severe oral disease. Children's oral disease may be legally prosecuted as a form of child neglect, and thus school officials assign a Child Protective Services (CPS) worker to monitor parents who are seen as refusing to comply with established standards of health or hygiene. Thus racialized public health practices contribute to the portrayal of the Central Valley as a space of potential disease contagion.

The conjoining of the threat of disease, racialized difference, and "illegality" create a border mentality among Mendota's public health professionals and educators. They perceive themselves as literally besieged by foreign health behaviors among a transient, rapidly changing population. This can be seen in the city's WIC office, on the wall of which hangs a poster – akin to a police suspect profile – with pictures of various "wanted" Mexican-origin tamarind candies with high lead content. Explaining the poster, a WIC worker said that she attended a WIC meeting in San Diego and the group took a fieldtrip across the border to see the substandard factories where these candies were manufactured. "Those kids, they run around eating [those candies] all the time. And then they come over here and bring them over here," she said. Her coworker, standing nearby, affirmed: "These kids eat a lot of candies from Mexico. . . . The problem is the candies easily come across the border, and they're made in plants where they don't have the regulations we have. So that poses a health risk." As this chapter will reveal, despite its location in the U.S.' interior, health professionals portray the Valley as a borderland – a space invaded by alien products where the presence of internal "foreigners" places national, social, and hygienic boundaries at constant risk.

Hygiene, foreign bodies, and governance

Hygiene, with its connotations of civilization and morality, has long served as a yardstick against which nonwhites' "fitness" for citizenship has been assessed. Negative portrayals of minority women's caregiving practices have long assumed a central place in both nativist and colonial discourses, in turn justifying whites' superior status throughout the world. When the Philippines was a U.S. colony, for example, public health officials' portrayals of Filipinas' unhygienic caregiving practices justified Filipinos' continued status as wards of the state. As Bonnie McElhinny (2005) writes, a purportedly "benevolent" campaign against high rates of infant mortality in the early 20th century strategically transformed Filipinas' mothering strategies into an argument for the continuation of the U.S.'s "civilizing influence." Meanwhile, on U.S. soil, the high infant mortality rate of Mexican-origin children in southern California led to stereotypes of Mexican immigrant women as "bad mothers" (Molina, 2006). These concerns cast U.S. public health departments as legitimate "stewards," portraying Mexicans as "stubborn children – a whole population who needed to be overseen, trained, controlled" (Molina, 2006, p. 74). In short, national and imperial projects have long aimed to transform subaltern practices of mothering, even as negative portrayals of such mothers in turn legitimized the states' authority and control.

New social histories of the role of public health in the American West reveal the centrality of hygiene to eugenic mechanisms of racial exclusion during the nation's first major wave of immigration between 1880 and 1920. Indeed, because of the high proportion of non-European immigrants, the relationship between public health promotion and nation-building may have been particularly virulent in California. On San Francisco's Angel Island, medical screenings were more intensive for Chinese, Filipino, and South Indian immigrants than those to which southern and eastern European immigrants were subjected to on the East coast. Meanwhile, at the U.S.–Mexico border, U.S. Public Health Service disinfection plants outlasted the threat of typhus that had initially spawned them, creating a regime of "eugenic gatekeeping" and enforced views of Mexicans as biologically inferior (Stern, 2005, pp. 58–59).[2] As Alexandra Stern writes, such medical inspection plants laid the foundation for the modern Border Patrol, and they helped to mark Mexicans as outsiders who could be admitted to the U.S. "only if sanitized by the methods of modern science" (2005, p. 71). Thus early in the 20th century, public health authorities lent a scientific basis to exclusive immigration policies, helping produce racialized portrayals of different immigrant groups.

Hygiene remains a potent symbolic marker of racial difference today, and public health continues to justify the exclusion of certain groups on eugenic grounds (Bashford, 2004; Molina, 2006). Yet scholars argue that the "new public health" entails a fundamental revision of the relationship between the state and its citizens. The focus of public health promotion in industrialized nations, they suggest, has increasingly shifted from imposing coercive quarantines to reforms encouraging individual self-governance (Rose, 1999). Nikolas Rose argues that the contemporary strategies of governance specify "the subjects of rule in terms of certain norms of civilization, effecting a division between the civilized member of society and those lacking the capacity to exercise their citizenship" (Rose, 1993, p. 291). One form of the "capacity to exercise citizenship" valorized by advanced liberal societies is the daily attention to the minutiae of personal hygiene. The upholding of American standards of personal health and hygiene as a measure of one's citizenship draws attention to new arrivals whose norms of hygiene are perceived to be different. In her study of immigration authorities' reception of Cambodian refugees, for example, Aihwa Ong (1995, pp. 1245–1246) shows that the Department of State's "Facts of Life in the United States" handbook inordinately stresses personal hygiene, including the elimination of "personal body odors" through practices such as bathing, the use of deodorant, mouthwash, and the brushing of teeth. In an era in which immigrant groups are judged as "worthy" or "unworthy" of public benefits based upon assessments of their self-reliance and individual responsibility, the hygienic practices of immigrant families bear now perhaps an even greater than previously symbolic load as a marker of capacity for self-governance. Adherence to modern norms of hygiene has become a central criterion in health professionals' assessments of immigrant groups' "fitness" for citizenship, and in the demarcation between "sanitary citizens" and "unsanitary subjects" (Briggs & Mantini-Briggs, 2003).

Oral disease assumed a prominent place in health professionals' discourses in signifying immigrant parents' "backwardness" and thus incapacity for self-governance. The most common childhood illness, oral disease, is disproportionately concentrated among low-income children (USDHHS, 2000). While Latinos have higher rates of oral disease than any other ethnic group apart from Native Americans, farmworker children as a group have rates of early childhood caries that reach five times those for Latino children in general (Nurko, Aponte-Merced, Bradley, & Fox, 1998; Weinstein, Domoto, Wohlers, & Koday, 1992). Health professionals in Mendota encountered severe oral decay in their everyday contact with farmworker children, offending their senses of smell and sight. As one Head Start teacher said: "You see kids with all sorts of dental problems – with huge holes, or you can smell it when they open their mouth." Meanwhile, the elementary school's School Nurse added: "You see kids with big holes in their mouths. Or sometimes the ones who just came in from Mexico they just have pointed jags from the decay. I don't even know how they eat."

To health professionals in Mendota, then, Mexican immigrant children's high rates of oral disease amplified their status as "aliens," serving as a particularly visible sign of this population's "foreign-ness." Educators viewed children's early childhood caries as a sign of their parents' lack of familiarity with modern caregiving practices – such as oral hygiene and proper infant feeding techniques. One WIC educator said: "The problem is that parents don't brush their [children's] teeth. And they fill their bottles with juice – and a lot of times it's Tampico, Kool-Aid, Sunny Delight, sometimes soda. It's crazy the things they put in there." While this WIC educator suggested that parents' irresponsibility and ignorance of proper child-feeding habits was the cause of their children's oral disease, others directly implicated products brought from Mexico. "My concerns are that they put a lot of juice in their kids' bottle and the kids have it all day long. Or they have them on those honey-filled pacifiers that they bring from Mexico," she said. These statements portray Mexican immigrants as unschooled in modern hygienic practices, targeting Mexico in particular as the source of such "backward" practices. They point to the way that a Mexican origin itself is perceived as unmodern and unhygienic: hygienic competence becomes a proxy for immigrant status.

Unlike complex childhood illnesses such as anemia, obesity, and diabetes, oral disease carries with it what we call a "stain of backwardness" because it is imagined as easily preventable with modern scientific methods. As the first-ever Surgeon General's Report on oral health, released in 2000, describes, the discovery of fluoride as an effective preventive measure after World War Two – along with the understanding of dental caries and periodontal diseases as largely preventable bacterial infections – have "allowed most middle-aged and younger Americans [to] expect to retain their natural teeth over their lifetime" (USDHHS, 2000, p. 1). Yet against this triumphal narrative of biomedical advances, the authors state, "*not all* Americans are achieving the same degree of health" (2000: 1). The report outlines measures necessary to render the "American dream" of "liv[ing] well into old age . . . with a high quality of life" (USDHHS, 2000, p. 4) available to the marginal populations overlooked by advances in modern science. Like other "diseases of civilization" (Bodley, 2008), in the U.S., oral disease is the result of a modern diet and lifestyle. Because of modern improvements in oral hygiene practices, such as tooth brushing with fluoridated toothpaste and community water fluoridation, the pronounced oral disease among minority populations indicates their adaptation to a "modern" diet without their concomitantly rapid adoption of "modern" health behaviors or access to "modern" advancements such as fluoridated water. For this reason, their high rate of oral disease appears as a blight upon the promise of medicine – a haunting reminder of uncivilized health behaviors and social inequality – amid an otherwise modern environment.

In keeping with this view of children's oral disease as an atavistic and unnecessary affliction in a modern society, health officials in Mendota spoke of children's high rates of early childhood caries with particular emotion and vehemence. As one Head Start educator said with dismay: "The thing that really gets you is seeing those kids who have their front teeth falling off in pieces or who can barely talk because of their problems. And you wonder, how can that parent go to sleep at night knowing that their kid is in pain and it could be avoided?" As farmworker children were perceived as not benefiting from the advances of public health promotion achieved during the past half-century, their dental decay was viewed as a visible sign of backwardness. In particular, as this educator's quote indicates, the oral disease of Mexican-origin children is viewed as a "stain" on their parents' caregiving skills, signaling the unfitness for citizenship of such newly arrived "foreigners."

Health educators draw upon such norms of hygiene as a symbolic marker of the boundary between Mexico and the U.S., between "internal foreigner" and "American." Nutritional educators in the WIC program, for example, speak disparagingly about what they called the "deficits of knowledge" they encountered among their Mexico-born food coupon recipients. One WIC educator said: "Our job is to do a lot of educating because the immigrants from Mexico don't know this stuff." Another explained: "We have to spend a lot of time educating, a lot of time dealing with foreign beliefs . . . The Hispanic ones, they make a shake with a raw egg in it. I think it has Nesquik, a raw egg, and a banana. And you explain that it could have bacteria and hurt them and they say, 'well, I did it with my five kids and I never had any problems.' Like that means it's fine!"

Making sanitary citizens and "citizen consanguines"

An examination of the interactions between educators from early childhood development programs and immigrant parents reveals the role of experts in human conduct – WIC educators, Head Start teachers, and health care professionals – in teaching immigrant parents and children about their "place" in American society. Not only do public health professionals attempt to instill in immigrants the "self-mastery" necessary for participation in liberal governance, but they also help adapt immigrant newcomers to the racial hierarchies of the nation. As Aihwa Ong argues, biomedicine not only reforms immigrant bodies, but "is constitutive of the social, economic and juridical practices that socialize biopolitical subjects of the modern welfare state" (1995, p. 1244). Many families in the Central Valley contain undocumented parents and citizen children, since increased border enforcement in the past decade has led many formerly migrant families to settle permanently in the U.S. Families with mixed legal status are quite common. Thus, analysis of how health officials interact with undocumented parents and their children reveals the way that immigrant incorporation is influenced by the fault lines of both generation and legal status.

Organizations such as WIC and Head Start devote a great deal of their time to instructing parents in the American norms of childrearing. These organizations utilize the family as an instrument for teaching self-governance, encouraging parents' assumption of the responsibility of parenthood as a form of "active citizenship" (Rose, 1993, p. 296). Immigrant parents are asked to subject their feeding and hygienic practices to WIC's scrutiny in exchange for monthly food coupons; WIC educators and nutritionists examine children's height, weight, and hemoglobin levels, as well as their diet and tooth-brushing habits. At monthly parent meetings, Head Start educators host lectures on child development, the nutritional content of meals, and proper individual hygiene. Through WIC and Head Start, then, the state governs at a distance, utilizing educators' expertise to scrutinize and Americanize immigrants' child-rearing practices and to instill norms of self-discipline.

As during the first major wave of immigration, personal health and hygiene, the "yardsticks of Americanization" (Molina, 2006, p. 45), play a large role in these organizations' socialization of new immigrant families. WIC educators inquire about parents' child-related oral hygiene and feeding practices, and teach parents to clean infants' baby teeth with a clean, wet rag when they first emerge. They urge parents to "find a dental home" for their child by the age of one. Meanwhile, Head Start requires that parents secure a medical and dental screening for each child before their children are enrolled; parents are additionally required to treat any problems discovered within 90 days, or their children are kicked out of the program. Children "dry-brush" their teeth with a fluoride spray after each meal in order to adopt the practice as an everyday routine. Head Start bars children from bringing in their baby bottles, to encourage the weaning of children. Finally, to teach parents proper nutrition, parents – under the supervision of Head Start educators – are put in charge of designing the program's "healthy" lunch menu. Such organizations thus attempt to normalize the domestic space immigrant families inhabit, focusing on domestic hygiene as an "index of civilization" (McElhinny, 2005).

Many of the public health professionals in the area are themselves second- or third-generation Mexican American; thus, such professionals draw upon hygienic hierarchy to enforce social distance between themselves and the "recent arrivals." In discussing the practices of farmworker parents, then, health professionals engage in a "geography of blame" (Farmer, 1993) that pinpoints Mexico as the source of unhealthy behaviors. In fingering Mexican practices as the culprit, this "geography of blame" ignores the American origins of the cariogenic diet – one high in fermentable carbohydrates and sugars – responsible for farmworker children's poor oral health while downplaying the structural issues that militate against farmworker children's health. Many immigrant parents were unprepared for the oral health implications of this diet as they came from rural areas dependent on subsistence farming, where they enjoyed a low incidence of oral disease despite few preventive oral health behaviors or state interventions.

While both WIC and Head Start attempt to instill in young citizens the norms of self-discipline through the institution of the family, they simultaneously inculcate different expectations of citizenship among parents and children. On the one hand, undocumented parents gain access to limited services through such programs due to their status as parents of citizen children. For example, while citizens are eligible for MediCal, California's public health insurance program, their undocumented immediate family is eligible for emergency MediCal because of their relation to such citizen children. While these programs prepare immigrant children to assume the rights and responsibilities of citizenship, the limited benefits they extend to their immigrant parents reflect their provisional membership in the social body. Undocumented parents live the contradiction in social rights open to themselves and their citizen children every day. While a majority of the parents we interviewed suffered from untreated dental pain or visible decay, they were asked to take their citizen children for dental visits at the behest of Head Start or the school system. Thus, what we call their "citizen consanguinity" placed undocumented immigrants in a unique relationship to the state.

Not all parents were fortunate enough to have access to the resources to demonstrate their "sanitary citizenship" – not even for their citizen children. Farmworker families' low incomes and fluctuating eligibility for California's dental Medicaid program (Denti-Cal), due to the seasonal nature of their work, restrict regular and preventive dental checkups. A shortage of dental health professionals to serve rural areas further limits access to dental care (Barker & Horton, 2008). Moreover, the "illegal" status of some farmworkers' children dramatically shaped parents' abilities to meet such norms. Undocumented children were not eligible for state-provided health care, while undocumented siblings of citizens were limited to emergency MediCal, which covers only the extractions, rather than restorations, of decayed teeth. While undocumented siblings gain a modicum of care due to their citizen consanguinity, it is bare-bones care limited to emergency treatment. In short, farmworker children's limited access to insurance and to dental treatment makes it difficult for them to comply with health educators' recommendations. Like other members of minority groups, farmworker parents are held to standards of hygiene which their unequal living conditions – which educators either ignore or overlook – preclude them from attaining (see also Molina, 2006; Shah, 2001).

Resisting the public health agenda

Not all parents subscribed to this new gospel of hygiene, however. One immigrant mother, for example, resisted subsequent dental visits for her children because she saw it as a form of imposed state discipline with few beneficial effects; her child's first trip to the dentist – required by Head Start – had been traumatic and left his cheek swollen. Because parents of undocumented children often wish to avoid the premature extractions the dentists suggest to resolve their children's oral disease, they may postpone treatment, hoping they will be able to eventually pay for restorations. This was in part the case for Mrs. Madrigal. In the meantime, however, such parents and their children continue to draw the disciplinary gaze of the school district, labeled "unsanitary subjects" due to their "noncompliance" with hygienic standards.

Yet even some parents of children who were citizens and therefore did have access to dental insurance were leery of the state's recommendations. Many immigrant farm-working parents – themselves from rural farming towns in Mexico – had experienced little decay themselves as children because of their relatively non-cariogenic diet – one based primarily on the crops of beans, corn, and squash that they grew. As poor subsistence farmers, most immigrant parents reported that their own parents rarely were able to afford to buy treats such as sodas and candy when they were children in Mexico (Horton & Barker, 2010). Yet upon arrival in the U.S., such parents often found that their own children – sometimes raised on baby bottles and in an environment in which soda and candy were plentiful – often had severe dental decay by the age of five. Because they not only were unfamiliar with the need for professional dentistry but also had little direct experience with dental restorations and anesthesia in their homelands, immigrant parents were understandably skeptical of professional dental treatment's benefits. Indeed, several spoke of dental treatment as a practice that placed their children at physical risk, often left them in pain, and sometimes left behind indelible markings.

In fact, the fall I began my fieldwork, a four-year-old Latino girl, Sherral Magaña, died in the nearby town of Hanford after what the clinic supervisor said was a severe allergic reaction to general anesthesia during a dental procedure. Frustrated that the dentist himself had not answered their questions about what had happened, and angry that the police were not prosecuting the dentist for medical malpractice, dozens of angry family members protested outside the dentist's offices, holding up signs reading YOU KILLED AN ANGEL and *PREGUNTAS Y NO RESPUESTAS* (Questions and No Answers) (Yale, 2005a, 2005b). The protest revealed the sentiment among this Latino immigrant family that the dental professionals and law-enforcement authorities were not taking the child's death seriously, perhaps as an indication of the lesser regard they held for the well-being of Latino families. Moreover, as news about the four-year-old's death spread, it only further fueled immigrant parents' doubts in both professional dental treatment and the wisdom of the school districts and Head Starts that required it.

For example, when I asked one immigrant mother about her child's oral health, she angrily opened her four-year-old daughter's mouth to show me a white patch, much like a blister marking the inside of the girl's cheek, a patch which had appeared two days after her dental appointment. "That's why we're afraid to take our kids to the dentist," she said. When I asked what had happened, the mother blamed the child's reaction on the local anesthesia. "It burned her," the mother explained. She further complained that when she had scheduled a follow-up appointment to have the dentist inspect her daughter's mouth, the dentist failed to explain the cause of the girl's blemish. When I asked this mother whether she had brought the child to the dentist at the Head Start's behest, she shushed my inquiry with an impatient shake of her head. "And the schools think we don't care about our children," she said. Thus, some immigrant parents resisted school officials' paternalism in assuming they knew what was best for their children. They rejected the schools' emphasis on hygiene as a marker of "enlightened" modern citizenship, instead portraying the dental treatment they required as unspeakably uncivilized.

Indeed, parents often negatively compared the quality of the treatment offered by the three dentists in town – only one of whom treated children under five, and none of whom offered general anesthesia – to the quality of dentists in Fresno, the nearest large city. When they could, immigrant parents often drove their children to Fresno, a 40-minute drive, to take them to private dentists who specialized in treating difficult-to-treat children. While they interpreted their poor treatment at the hands of local dentists as an interpersonal affront, they felt themselves the victims of a broader geographical insult as well. "The dentists are no good here," explained one immigrant father when his child's filling fell out the day after it had been placed. The perceived low quality of dental treatment in the area – perhaps a reflection of its being a rural, dentally underserved area – only exacerbated immigrant parents' mistrust of professional dental practice.

Parents particularly objected to the practices of the one dentist in Mendota, Dr. Bishop, who did treat children under five years old and did accept MediCal. Dr. Bishop, in turn, said he began practicing in Mendota right after he graduated from dental school because rents were cheap and he "could not afford to go anywhere else." They reported that Dr. Bishop – who had practiced in the area for more than 18 years and did not speak Spanish – often extracted children's teeth rather than restoring them. Moreover, they reported that he often immobilized children during treatment by strapping them to a board without parents' informed consent. Restraining children in this manner is one of eight possible techniques to manage the behavior of children deemed "difficult-to-treat" because of their young age or because of their extensive decay. Yet studies frequently show that parents universally deem this practice far less acceptable than that of providing local or general anesthesia or actively restraining children (Eaton, McTigue, Fields, & Beck, 2005). Immobilizing children by strapping them to a papoose board requires the consent of parents (AAPD, 2015) – an issue complicated by the language gap between many immigrant parents and many dentists who did not speak Spanish.

One immigrant mother from Jalisco, Mrs. Sandoval, for example, told me of her experience with Dr. Bishop. She said that her 10-year-old son has badly decayed molars. Several years ago, she drove two hours to take her son to a pedodontist in the town of Hanford; the pedodontist was able to perform fillings on the child's molars under sedation. She said she was very happy with that experience. More recently, however, she took her 10-year-old to Dr. Bishop in Mendota. Before her son was ushered into the treatment room, a bilingual secretary asked Mrs. Sandoval to sign a piece of paper in English that she could not read. When Mrs. Sandoval arose to accompany her son into the treatment room, the secretary informed her that the paperwork she had signed bound her to remaining in the waiting room while Dr. Bishop treated her son. When her son emerged, Mrs. Sandoval was alarmed to find that he was speechless; she says he began crying when he got home. Her son told her that Dr. Bishop had strapped him down. "As though he were an animal," she said. In short, immigrant parents spoke of the barbarity of the dental treatment their children received – in the form of accidental burns, premature extractions, and forcible strappings – as substandard treatment communicating their status as second-class citizens.

Not only did the traumatic experience of Mrs. Sandoval's son enrage Mrs. Sandoval; she was also equally angry that Dr. Bishop did not meaningfully ask her for her permission before strapping her son down. To Mrs. Sandoval, then, Dr. Bishop's office's preemption of the informed consent process treated parents who are monolingual in Spanish as though they were judgmentally impaired and incapable of reason. To Mrs. Sandoval, this practice explicitly communicated to parents that they were in fact second-class citizens. "Why do they have such bad dentists in this area? They think the people are ignorant and can't speak English so they won't protest," she said. Similarly, a Head Start nurse said of Dr. Bishop, "Some people, like this guy – they think they can get away with it because people don't have papers so what are they going to do." Thus, while many immigrant parents interpreted rude interactions with secretaries and dentists as an interpersonal slight, they viewed the poor quality of dentists in the area as a matter of systemic racial and legal discrimination. Parents like Mrs. Sandoval viewed the abuses they experienced at the hands of dentists in the area as marker of their inhabiting an internal borderlands of sorts – one in which substandard dental practices predominated. They viewed the poor treatment their children received at the hands of local dentists, and such dentists' dismissal of their authority as parents, as an index of their low social standing in both the area and in the nation.

Conclusion

This chapter serves as a cautionary tale about the racialized implications of public health promotion programs in internal borderlands spaces. In public health circles, the persistence of poor oral health among low-income populations is perceived as what we call a "stain of backwardness," a deplorable sign in an otherwise modern society. To public health officials, Mexican immigrants' lack of familiarity with preventive oral hygiene practices and their children's decayed teeth amplify their status as "aliens" and visibly symbolize their "foreign-ness." Yet public health promotion programs must take into account the structural barriers that prevent immigrant parents from complying with "American" norms of hygiene, and must instill health educators with a sensitivity to the fact that the norms of caregiving they advocate are in fact culturally constructed adaptations to an "American" diet.

Public health experts must also critically scrutinize the role programs play in portrayals of minority populations. Public health officials have historically fixated on different health issues among minority populations at different historical moments, each one speaking to a specific racial anxiety. The focus on Latino children's oral hygiene recalls public health concerns regnant during the first great wave of immigration, when cleanliness was infused with morality and patriotism and served as an index of Americanization (Molina, 2006; Shah, 2001). Deployed by public health educators in a neoliberal era, proper personal and familial hygiene carries an ever-new moral significance – that of capacity for self-governance. In short, the high rates of oral disease among Mexican-origin children are seen to reflect poorly upon their parents. Critical analyses of public health campaigns in colonial and postcolonial settings will allow public health officials to be mindful of the relations of power these campaigns create, and the broader role they play in the discursive construction of minority groups' "fitness" for inclusion in the body politic.

Editor commentary

Sarah Horton and Judith Barker's work with immigrant communities along the California–Mexico border reveals the pervasive nature of public health politics. Drawing on Brigg and Mantini Brigg's constructs of *unsanitary subjects* and *sanitary citizens*, they describe the *biopolitical* nature of oral hygiene (and hygiene- and sanitation-related public health efforts more generally) in defining norms and setting behavioral standards for inclusion into the body politic.

In addition, they identify the following:

- The introduction of the "new public health" drive toward responsibilization, which has shifted the relationship between citizen and state from one of coercion and quarantine to one of self-governance.
- Hygiene as historical and uniquely American, the measure of civilization and morality.
- The use of schools and other non-health institutions, to provide a disciplinary gaze, in a process of *governance at a distance*.
- *Geographies of blame* that pinpoint certain locations as culprits for bad health, disregarding social, political, and economic inequalities that afford differential access to health technologies and resources, both in particular locations and by different populations within shared geographies.
- Resistance to health policies as an objection to imposed state discipline; substandard treatment resulting from ethnicity and economic status; paternalism of school officials; and the positioning of English-speaking, educated professionals as superior to Spanish-speaking immigrants in determining what is appropriate childcare and what are rational health behaviors.

Notes

1 To protect the confidentiality of our interviewees, all names in this article are pseudonyms.

2 Historian Alexandra Minna Stern (1999, 2005) describes how the U.S. Public Health Service's disinfection plant on the border between El Paso and Ciudad Juárez enforced inspection procedures more strenuous than those to which Eastern European immigrants were subjected at Ellis Island. After a minor outbreak of typhus fever in Mexico in 1916, the plant was enlisted to enforce a medical quarantine. All those crossing the border were stripped naked, bathed, deloused, their hair shorn and their clothes sterilized; they were also forced to pass, naked, in front of medical inspectors to be assayed for physical and mental defects. She describes how Mexican immigrants' forced nudity and disinfection continued well into the 1920s, long after the threat of typhus had subsided (Stern, 1999, pp. 41–49).

References

AAPD. (2015). Guideline on Behavior Guidance for the Pediatric Dental Patient. American Association of Pediatric Dentistry. *Clinical Practice Guidelines Reference Manual, 37*(6), 180–193.

Aguirre International. (2005). The California Farm Labor Force: Overview and Trends from the National Agricultural Workers Study. Retrieved from http://agcenter.ucdavis.edu/documents/CalifFarmLaborForceNAWS.pdf.

Barker, J. C., & Horton, S. B. (2008). An ethnographic study of Latino preschool children's oral health in rural California: Intersections among family, community, provider, and regulatory sectors. *BMC Oral Health, 8*(1), 8.

Bashford, A. (2004). *Imperial Hygiene: A Critical History of Colonialism, Nationalism, and Public Health*. New York: Palgrave Macmillan.

Bodley, J. (2008). *Victims of Progress*. Walnut Creek: Altamira Press.

Briggs, C. L., & Mantini-Briggs, C. (2003). *Stories in the Time of Cholera: Racial Profiling During a Medical Nightmare.* Berkeley: University of California Press.

Eaton, J. J., McTigue, D. J., Fields, H. W., & Beck, M. F. (2005). Attitudes of contemporary parents toward behavior management techniques used in pediatric dentistry. *Pediatric Dentistry, 27*(2), 107–113.

Farmer, P. (1993). *AIDS and Accusation: Haiti and the Geography of Blame.* Berkeley: University of California Press.

Gonzales, R., & McChesney, J. (2002, November 11–14). California's Central Valley: NPR series profiles the state's backstage rural breadbasket. *National Public Radio.*

Horton, S. B., & Barker, J. C. (2010). Stigmatized biologies: Examining the cumulative effects of oral health disparities for Mexican American children. *Medical Anthropology Quarterly, 24*(2), 199–219.

McElhinny, B. (2005). "Kissing a baby is not at all good for him:" Infant mortality, medicine, and colonial modernity in the U.S.-occupied Philippines. *American Anthropologist, 107*(2), 183–194.

Molina, N. (2006). *Fit to Be Citizens? Public Health and Race in Los Angeles, 1879–1939.* Berkeley: University of California Press.

Ngai, M. M. (2004). *Impossible Subjects: Illegal Aliens and the Making of Modern America.* Princeton: Princeton University Press.

Nurko, C., Aponte-Merced, L., Bradley, E. L., & Fox, L. (1998). Dental caries prevalence and dental health care of Mexican-American workers' children. *ASCD Journal of Dentistry for Children, 65*(1):65–72.

Ong, A. (1995). Making the biopolitical subject: Cambodian immigrants, refugee medicine and cultural citizenship in California. *Social Science & Medicine, 40*(9), 1243–1257.

Ong, A. (1996). Cultural citizenship as subject-making: Immigrants negotiate racial and cultural boundaries in the United States. *Current Anthropology, 37*(5), 737–762.

Rose, N. (1993). Government, authority, and expertise in advanced liberalism. *Economy and Society, 22*(3), 283–299.

Rose, N. (1999). *Powers of Freedom: Reframing Political Thought.* Cambridge, UK: Cambridge University Press.

Shah, N. (2001). *Contagious Divides: Epidemics and Race in San Francisco's Chinatown.* Berkeley, CA: University of California Press.

Stern, A. M. (1999). Buildings, boundaries, and blood: Medicalization and nation-building on the U.S.–Mexico border, 1910–1930. *Hispanic American Historical Review, 79*(1), 41–81.

Stern, A. M. (2005). *Eugenic Nation: Faults and Frontiers of Better Breeding in Modern America.* Berkeley, CA: University of California Press.

U.S. Census Bureau. 2010. United States Census 2010. Retrieved from: http://www.census.gov/2010census/.

USDHHS. (2000). Oral Health in America: A Report of the Surgeon General. Rockville, MD: U.S. Department of Health and Human Services, National Institute of Dental and Craniofacial Research, National Institutes of Health.

Weinstein, P., Domoto, P., Wohlers, K., & Koday, M. (1992). Mexican-American parents with children at risk for baby bottle tooth decay: Pilot study at a migrant farmworkers clinic. *ASCD Journal of Dentistry for Children, 59*(5), 376–383.

Yale, S. (2005a). Family of Girl Who Died During Dental Procedure Gather to Demand Answers. *Hanford Sentinel.* Retrieved from http://hanfordsentinel.com/breaking_news/family-of-girl-who-died-following-dental-procedure-gather-to/article_761593af-4e19-5d12-bf8d-8de970df9dad.html

Yale, S. (2005b). Girl, 4, Dies After Dental Procedure. *Hanford Sentinel.* Retrieved from http://hanfordsentinel.com/front/girl-dies-after-dental-procedure/article_2a2eb85b-5a5c-5da5-a593-3ad7da61a6e6.html

8

DRUG PATENTS AND SHIT POLITICS IN SOUTH AFRICA

Refiguring the Politics of the 'Scientific' and the 'Global' in Global Health Interventions

Christopher J. Colvin and Steven Robins

Introduction

In most accounts of the history of AIDS activism in South Africa, the case of AIDS denialism and the fight against the expansion of antiretroviral therapy (ART) stands out as the signature South African case of local resistance to global public health intervention. The 'global' in this case refers to an international alliance of global health institutions, donor countries, development programs, and a broad network of health activists and medical practitioners – inspired and coordinated locally by the most important post-apartheid social movement, the Treatment Action Campaign (TAC). The TAC demanded access to ART for those in the global South who could not afford this lifesaving treatment (Colvin & Robins, 2014; Mbali, 2013; Nattrass, 2007). To many observers, the TAC, along with its national and global allies, had a singular focus and demand at the heart of its campaign – as one commentator has put it plainly but aptly, getting 'drugs into bodies' (Smith & Siplon, 2006).

Resisting this push for biomedical treatment of HIV were global 'AIDS denialists' and 'dissidents,' led locally by President Mbeki, his Health Minister, and a range of allies who worked to thwart attempts to impose 'Northern' biomedical solutions to 'African' problems (Kalichman, 2009; Nattrass, 2007; Rasnik, 2005). Denialists argued that large U.S. and European drug companies were promoting antiretroviral medications they secretly knew to be toxic as a way to profit from the suffering of those living with HIV in southern Africa and elsewhere. They also argued that a focus on drug technology was implicitly a way to "pharmaceuticalize" (Biehl, 2007) poverty and ignore persisting social, economic, and political inequalities, both local and global, that drove public health crises. They instead lobbied for the development of 'local' solutions, to be drawn from a combination of indigenous African scientific and traditional sources of knowledge.

This is a fascinating moment in the history of South African health politics, one that raises a number of critical questions about how and why AIDS denialism found traction in South Africa, both within the highest offices of the state and the most local of community-based organizations. Like many of the cases reviewed in this volume, the reasons for this resistance included ambivalent citizen–state relationships, suspicions about economic and political globalization, conflicting epistemologies of disease and healing technologies, and a perceived disconnect between the proposed biomedical solutions and the lived and embodied experiences of those bearing the brunt of the epidemic (Colvin, 2012; Kalichman, 2009; Kenyon, 2008; Nattrass, 2010).

In this chapter, our interests in local resistance to global biomedical discourse and practice specifically relate to approaches to public health maintenance. Rather than examining outright resistance to the imposition of external biomedical interventions – as in AIDS denialism – we consider two cases where local communities and health activists have instead demanded global intervention but resisted the ways in which those interventions have conventionally been implemented. In doing so, we hope to expand the ways that 'local' resistance to the 'global' can be understood and illustrate how the political consequences of the 'scientific' and the 'global' can be challenged without renouncing aspirations for the benefits of scientific knowledge or global interconnection.

The arguments in this chapter emerge from the experiences of two significant health social movements in South Africa – the above-mentioned fight for access to ART, and the recent 'shit politics' (Robins, 2014a) that has coalesced around local struggles to improve sanitation and security in the country's poorest communities. Using this material, we develop two key arguments in the chapter. First, these movements have worked to refigure the typical relationships between science and politics by embracing a conventional 'science-as-truth' view of the world but challenging the social, economic, and political inequalities that too often both support and result from the application of this model in practice. They have questioned not science itself, but the use of the 'scientific' as a way to entrench social and political hierarchies.

Second, these movements have worked to refigure the relationships between the global and the political by affirming the importance of local context when implementing interventions but challenging the notion that local solutions need to be 'locally appropriate' and 'sustainable.' These terms, they argue, are too often defined by others, and mask a diluting of global technologies, rights and resources and a defense of status quo notions of what is feasible in the global South. These movements have instead demanded access to 'what they have' in the North, challenging straightforward appeals to difference of the local and asserting a right of access to a universal 'global standard.'

Refiguring the Politics of Science

Treatment Action Campaign

South Africa's Treatment Action Campaign (TAC) was established in 1998 in reaction to the national government's weak, fragmented, and ineffective response to the HIV epidemic up to that point. Its early membership was comprised largely of anti-apartheid and gay rights activists based in Cape Town, but the movement grew quickly into a broad-based coalition of activists, public health and medical practitioners, and community members from both rural and urban settings and across the class spectrum (Geffen, 2010; Mbali, 2013). TAC began campaigning for a more committed fight against HIV across the health system, with an early focus on ensuring access to medication for prevention of mother-to-child transmission in the public sector health services (Nattrass, 2007; Yamin & Gloppen, 2011). Activists were also concerned about the exorbitant prices that Northern pharmaceutical companies were charging for antiretroviral medicines (ARVs) as well as the dramatic levels of HIV-related stigma and discrimination that persisted in both communities and public health facilities (Heywood, 2009).

Since its inception, TAC's work has been characterized by its defense of the mainstream scientific consensus around the cause, prevention, and treatment of HIV – over and against the government's lengthy infatuation with AIDS denialism – and its close working relationships with academic experts in medicine, public health, law, and the social sciences. This defense of the scientific view of HIV and the necessary biomedical response, however, was also always accompanied by an effort to put science to its own political ends and work against the many ways in which conventional scientific discourse and practice depends on and perpetuates social and economic inequalities.

For example, during one of its first high-profile legal challenges against drug company pricing, TAC faced considerable difficulties in understanding and mobilizing the complex legal, economic, and scientific arguments around the development, distribution, pricing, and pharmacology of ARVs that were at stake in the trial. TAC enlisted the help of biomedical researchers, clinicians, health systems experts, and health economists, both in South Africa and abroad, in drafting the affidavits it needed for the case (Colvin & Heywood, 2012). This support was extensive and in-depth, and proved critical in securing a positive outcome in the trial. It also cemented a range of relationships between TAC and individual researchers and institutions, relationships TAC would continue to draw on as it continued its legal and political work to secure access to ART (Ahmad, 2013).

Rather than allowing its engagement with scientific expertise to remain a narrow aspect of its legal strategies, however, TAC also worked from the beginning to bring this knowledge to its own membership. During the trial described above, TAC spent a great deal of time educating its members and its key political and media allies about HIV, ART, and the specific issues at stake in the case. This effort included workshops with overseas activists and experts as well as all-night vigils to work through the scientific, political, and legal issues at stake. TAC also made all of the court papers readily accessible on their website as soon as they were available, including a series of technical affidavits submitted by the drug companies that provided key insights into heretofore hidden drug-company pricing practices (Colvin & Heywood, 2012).

TAC also took its engagement with the technical aspects of HIV and ART provision beyond the legal context and developed it as a signature feature of its grassroots activism. One of the more distinctive features of TAC's overall political strategy has been the development of its 'treatment literacy practitioner' (TLP) model (Robins, 2009), a kind of 'expert patient' (Kielmann & Cataldo, 2010) meant to bring detailed technical knowledge of HIV and its treatment to the level of individual patients. TLPs were trained to counsel people with HIV on both the nature and progression of HIV disease itself as well as the form and function of the different antiretroviral (ARV) medications and the ways in which each disrupted different parts of the viral life cycle. This instruction was remarkably detailed, with patients learning about different aspects of the immune system, viral pathogenesis, and the mechanisms of each type of ARV. They were encouraged to learn the scientific names of the drugs as well as the approved first- and second-line regimens, dosages, and potential side effects. Speaking at a conference, Vuyiseka Dubula, General Secretary of TAC, explained:

> So the first thing we did, we empowered ourselves with knowledge. You know your facts. You are going to be challenging doctors, you are going to be challenging nurses, you are going to be challenging government, you are going to be challenging politicians and the international community. So if you don't know your story, it is easy for them to throw you out of the boardroom. (Quoted in the film *Taking HAART*) (Lewis, 2011).

Finally, like the generation of AIDS activists who preceded them in North America, TAC activists have taken a leading role in advocating for safe but rapid technological development of more effective drugs with fewer side effects and swift regulatory approval and distribution of these drugs (Epstein, 1996; Geffen, 2010; Nattrass, 2012). Through their networks in research and clinical practice, they have stayed abreast of the latest developments and opportunities in HIV prevention and treatment and learned in detail about the legal and research processes required to develop, test, and implement new drugs. One can see this focus on mobilizing detailed knowledge most dramatically in the shape of their press releases, many of which run for several pages, outlining and explaining in plain language specific scientific, legal, and other technical issues at stake and providing considerable references and further resources. This approach involves more than just a rhetorical reference to the scientific as a way to buttress their claims (though that may also be at play); it also involves a sustained and serious effort to educate its membership and the public more broadly, and in turn mobilize that new awareness into focused political action.

The Social Justice Coalition

The Social Justice Coalition (SJC) has employed similar strategies in its efforts to improve sanitation and security in Cape Town townships. SJC was founded in 2008 in the aftermath of xenophobic violence that erupted in South African cities. The organization established itself in an informal settlement in Khayelitsha (RR Section).

It focuses efforts on the intersection of inadequate sanitation and everyday violence and insecurity. Despite the fact that poor services and lack of safety were part of people's daily lives in RR Section, SJC's immediate challenge was how to render these everyday realities of poor sanitation and violence politically legible. Activists recalled how difficult it was initially to make residents of RR Section view daily experiences of children playing in raw sewage that ran through streets and into shacks as politically unacceptable. By means of door-to-door sanitation literacy programs – not unlike TAC's treatment literacy approach – SJC activists were ultimately able to challenge this normalized reality and transform sanitation into a politically legible matter of public concern and citizen rights.

There are historical reasons why human waste has seldom been considered to be a properly political and public matter. Prior to the 16th century in Europe, human waste was usually dumped in the streets, fields, or rivers. Then, in 1539, an ordinance was introduced in France that required that human waste be stored in the basement of houses. In his aptly titled book, *The History of Shit*, Dominique Laporte (2000) notes that France's royal decree of 1539 required that "every individual or individual family hold on to personal waste before carrying it out of the city." France's decree of 1539 is one of countless sanitary laws that have been introduced by states throughout the world. This privatization and domestication of human waste still has consequences today.

Yet, political theorists and commentators have generally shied away from engaging with the political dimensions of human waste. For European political theorists of democracy such as Hannah Arendt (1958), the private domain of the household (the *oikos*), and everything that takes place within its walls, was not considered to be a properly political matter of public concern. For Arendt, a fiercely masculinist thinker, 'proper politics' consisted of debate and deliberation on public matters beyond the feminized domestic realm; private household matters such as defecation, toilets, and sanitation did not qualify as 'political.'

Historically constituted obstacles may prevent such private matters from entering the domain of public debate and deliberative democracy. For instance, long histories of stigma and shame associated with excrement and open defecation, especially among the poor, have ensured that these matters are only gradually becoming part of what Arjun Appadurai (2002) and others refer to as a "politics of s★★★" that is emerging in Asia. In a book entitled *Shit Matters*, Lyla Mehta (2011) writes about how Community-Led Total Sanitation Programs, emerging out of Bangladesh, have opened up such debates in rural villages, thereby challenging the silence and normalization of abysmal sanitation conditions in many parts of the developing world. Clearly, shit can become political.

Even so, sanitation and politics have always been intertwined, despite being framed by bureaucrats as purely apolitical and technical matters of urban infrastructure, planning, and public health. In colonial Africa, as well as apartheid South Africa, states have used sanitary and hygiene laws to displace the poor from the middle-class city centers and suburbs to the urban margins. Numerous poor and working-class neighborhoods such as District Six in Cape Town, South Africa, have been demolished in the name of hygiene, sanitation, and public health. There are many examples of people using their bodily waste as a weapon in a struggle for political recognition (the Cape Town example is explained below) (see Robins, 2014b). Such efforts suggest that bodily fluids and functions such as defecation, perhaps the most private and intimate of household activities, can, under certain conditions, enter the circuits of public debate and political life. As sanitation activists today observe, it is precisely the rape of women going to toilets at night that makes defecating in Cape Town's informal settlements and India's rural villages so dangerous and political. It is also women who have to deal with the dire health consequences of children playing in spaces contaminated by raw sewage.

Addressing these intertwined public concerns and citizen rights around sanitation and safety issues at the level of the state required strategic use of a kind of 'slow activism,' a critical engagement with bureaucratic logic and technical expertise (Nixon, 2011; Robins, 2014a, 2014c). For instance, in an effort to render these conditions legible to the state, the wider public, and those who suffer these conditions on a daily basis, SJC commissioned, translated, and disseminated scientific research that documented the *E. coli* levels in RR Section that demonstrated the high risk of disease from exposure to water contaminated by raw sewage (Social Justice Coalition, 2010).

SJC also waged an ongoing battle to persuade city officials to accept that large numbers of people living in the City of Cape Town did not have access to basic sanitation. According to SJC, the City was using outdated and inaccurate census data to justify its distribution of public services, especially in 'informal settlements' that are often missed on censuses and grow at rapid rates. Rather than simply arguing that the City's data were inaccurate, SJC eventually conducted its own audit of the number of people living there as well as the social services available and provided this data both to the City and to the public at large (Social Justice Coalition, 2013). Finally, SJC has also regularly made use of student researchers and university-based academics to support a process of ongoing knowledge production relevant to the issues at stake.

SJC's engagement with matters of safety and sanitation thus involved a repertoire of tactics that included the use of statistics, qualitative research, litigation, the media, personal testimonies, and protests. Like TAC, they have been careful to integrate their engagement with scientific expertise into the other components of their activism in order to achieve maximum political effect by, for example, widely publicizing the results of its social audit and capacitating its members to understand and engage with this material. They have also been able to get a number of medical researchers and professors of public health and medicine, as well as social scientists such as the author, to write feature articles in local and national press on SJC and conditions in Cape Town's informal settlements.

These methods were also used to make the City of Cape Town more accountable and transparent in its delivery of policing services, culminating in SJC's successful establishment of the Pikoli and O'Reagan Commission of Inquiry into Policing in Khayelitsha. Like TAC's engagement with health professionals and medical scientists and researchers, SJC mobilized criminologists, NGOs, and various other crime and policing experts to analyze crime statistics in order to identify the distribution of different forms of crime in Khayelitsha. For instance, an analysis of statistics from RR Section revealed that crime figures on gender-based violence were dramatically underreported. This was attributed to the fact that courts and police were overburdened, and only homicide was being routinely reported to the police. The commission's findings were also used to draw attention to resource and infrastructure disparities in policing in Cape Town. Like the social audits documenting disparities in sanitation, SJC was able to use the commission of inquiry findings to show how poor neighborhoods in Khayelitsha had vastly less policing resources than the much wealthier, historically white, suburbs.

SJC's engagement with scientific expertise, statistical data, testimonials, journalists, and researchers to lobby and pressure the state for resources mirrored the tactics of TAC (Robins, 2009). Their techniques of 'data-driven activism' (Lievrouw, 2011), combined with litigation and grassroots mobilization, does not indicate outright resistance to scientific logics and technical interventions, but neither does it signal acquiescence to the apolitical and technicist practices of state-sponsored science. Instead, it demonstrates a strategic engagement with the language and logic of science and the bureaucratic state *alongside* a critical political perspective, with a disruptive intent to mobilize their own counter-practices of 'active citizenship' and knowledge production. For both TAC and SJC, conventional science was mobilized but as a means to a different set of political ends, ones that would reduce rather than increase the inequalities that too often flow from technocratic interventions.

Refiguring the politics of the global and local

In this second half of the chapter, we examine another aspect of the AIDS and sanitation activism, this time involving the relationships at stake between the global and the local in these political struggles. Many political struggles over global public health initiatives, including the other case studies described in this volume, are rooted in a resistance to the imposition of global, and presumably universally effective and acceptable, interventions by Northern actors in ways that either ignore or actively denigrate local experience, perspectives, and contexts. This political problem is also present in some of the HIV and sanitation activism undertaken by TAC, SJC, and other organizations. For example, TAC has worked hard against the imposition of expert-driven, technicist medical interventions by introducing treatment literacy campaigns that empowered people living with AIDS. Similarly, SJC has argued that sanitation matters ought not to be simply left to the engineers and city officials, and ordinary citizens need to have at their disposal 'lay expert' knowledge that can empower them in their interactions with city officials and technocrats.

For the most part, however, AIDS and sanitation activists in South Africa have not been asking for 'locally appropriate' and 'sustainable' solutions. It is not that they have rejected the idea that interventions need to be locally appropriate or sustainable. Rather, they have resisted the implicit political logic that is carried within those terms, a logic that assumes poorer countries would not be able to afford and deliver 'First World' technology and that solutions need to be adapted – and expectations scaled down – in order to secure a comfortable fit with the 'local' context.

Resistance to global understandings of the (limits of the) local first appeared in South African AIDS activism in reaction to widely publicized claims by U.S. aid agency representatives that Africans were not good candidates for daily ART regimens, given their loose relationship with time and thus inability to take their medication on the required strict schedule (Herbert, 2001). A less overtly racist but similarly problematic claim came in the form of public health experts in the U.S. and Europe who believed that the provision of ART was too complex and burdensome a task for the struggling and overcrowded public sector health services in South Africa. These claims, that 'the local' would in fact prevent delivery of global/Northern technological salvation, became the catalyst for the 'pilot demonstration' project that TAC, Medicins Sans Frontieres (MSF), the University of Cape Town, and others developed in Cape Town in 2000 to deliver ART in public facilities to public sector patients with HIV (Stinson et al., 2014). The explicit goal of this project was to demonstrate to Northern donors and public health policymakers that an African public health system delivering ART to an economically marginalized population could achieve equal or even better outcomes than Northern medical services. TAC, MSF, and their partners were successful in this pilot and have since been consistent in their demands for public sector access to whatever the latest globally accepted standard of care is for HIV.

TAC and its allies took a similar approach when arguments about the affordability and cost-effectiveness of ART were raised as significant barriers to increasing access to ART. They did not accept the argument that ARVs at their current prices were unaffordable for even a middle-income country like South Africa. Instead, TAC not only carried out a conventional political and legal campaign for a reduction in the prices of these medicines, but also they worked with sociologists and health economists to demonstrate in rich technical detail how these medications were not only affordable, but would produce a net savings for the country (Nattrass, 2004). In challenging conventional framings of the affordability of global technology and the scarcity of local resources, they not only mobilized science effectively (as discussed in this chapter's first section), but also they developed a compelling case that access to the global standard was not only possible and morally right, but even cost effective.

In fact, most of the examples in the previous section describing TAC's efforts to mobilize scientific expertise to new political ends were also about ensuring local access to global technology and refusing to accept global discourses that local contexts, especially in Africa, might render ART unacceptable, impractical, or unaffordable. In a similar fashion, much of SJC's activism has been focused on insisting that people living in the poorest communities of Cape Town deserve access to the same basic infrastructure and services afforded the wealthier residents of the same city.

In this section, however, we want to highlight the case of another activist organization addressing issues of sanitation and health, but this time from a fairly different political perspective and strategy. The Ses'khona People's Rights Movement is based, like SJC, in the Cape Town township of Khayelitsha. This organization is more clearly organized around a rejection of conventional discourses and practices of public health intervention as well as the technocratic logic of the bureaucratic state. Even though Ses'khona's demands for improved sanitation infrastructure and services mirror those of SJC's, its more militant modes of activism are very different than the rational-scientific and deliberative democratic practices of SJC, TAC, MSF, and other similar activist organizations.

In the run-up to the 2011 local government elections, a group of African National Congress (ANC) activists, the same individuals who two years later founded Ses'khona, "discovered" open toilets in Makhaza informal settlement in Khayelitsha. These were conventional flush toilets that had been installed by the City outside of people's homes, but without any enclosing walls. These activists accused the Democratic Alliance–controlled (DA)[1] local and provincial government in the Western Cape of racism and violating the privacy and dignity of black South Africans and took the matter of the open toilets to the Human Rights Commission (HRC) and the Western Cape High Court.

When, in response to both the HRC finding and the court order, the provincial government attempted to enclose these toilets using corrugated iron, ANC activists tore down the enclosures and demanded "proper" brick structures. These political developments were widely reported in the media as the 'Toilet Elections' and the 'Toilet Wars.' A couple of months later the ANC was also politically compromised by the discovery of unenclosed toilets in a township in the ANC-run Free State Province. Meanwhile, in response to mounting pressure from the SJC's social audit findings of inadequate sanitation services in informal settlements as well as the open toilets scandal, the City of Cape Town began distributing thousands of portable flush toilets (PFTs) in settlements where, for various reasons, it was deemed unfeasible to provide conventional sanitation infrastructure. Some of the reasons put forward by the City of Cape Town included the high water table, illegally occupied land, high shack densities, and variety of other technical reasons.

In 2013, in response to the City's rollout of 'portaloos,' a group of community activists from Ses'khona began hurling portable toilet containers filled with feces on Cape Town's N2 highway, in the departures section of the Cape Town International Airport, on the steps of the provincial legislature, and at various other sites in the city. The activists insisted that there was a sanitation crisis in the informal settlements in Cape Town, and that the provision of portable toilets was totally unacceptable. The response of the City of Cape Town's DA politicians and senior officials was to deny that these 'portaloos' resembled the much maligned 'bucket toilets,' literally buckets of human waste that individuals transported to designated disposal areas. Instead, PFTs were described as safe, hygienic, properly sealed, water-based, and fully flushable. For their troubles, the leaders of the airport poo protests were arrested and charged under the Civil Aviation Act, and some were temporarily suspended by the ANC. These feces flingers from the urban periphery had literally dragged the stench of shit from the shantytowns to Cape Town's centers of political and economic power.

Sithembele Majova, an ANC branch chairperson and leader of the protests, complained that the DA's portable toilets "cause a smell in the houses" and that it is "unhygienic to live with poo inside the house." He added, "We want the people who are living in those nice [upper middle class] areas like Constantia to feel how poo can damage your life when it is next to you."[2] The Ses'khona leadership were outraged that the poor had to use these portable toilets in single-roomed tin shacks, as this meant that intimate partners, parents, and children had to relieve themselves in the same room, and the same space in which they slept, received guests, and prepared their meals.

The Ses'khona poo protests of 2013 signaled a rejection of the technocratic and bureaucratic rationalities of the state in favor of mass mobilization characterized by an affectively charged politics of the instant media spectacle (Robins, 2014a). At the same time, however, they made it clear that second- or third-class solutions to sanitation were not going to be acceptable in the poorer communities in Cape Town and demanded that these citizens be granted access to the same standards of sanitation and public infrastructure that was available in other parts of the city.

This rejection of substandard, intermediate, and temporary solutions mirrors similar rejections in other parts of the country of efforts to develop locally appropriate, technologically innovative, and sustainable solutions to sanitation and housing problems. These other contested interventions include self-composting toilets promoted by the Gates Foundation and the 'iShack' solar energy project in Stellenbosch.

The Bill and Melinda Gates Foundation designated 3 million USD toward the 'Reinventing the Toilet' program. Officially launched in 2011, this program provides funding for researchers at eight universities, including the University of KwaZulu-Natal in Durban, to design a new toilet that is both appropriate for economic conditions in developing countries and reduces the environmental impact of flushable toilets. The idea is to provide people in the developing world (40% of the world's population) without access to reticulated water and sanitation systems cheap, waterless toilets that can turn human waste into clean water and agriculturally efficient byproducts (i.e., manure and fertilizer). But, these Gates-funded eco-friendly urine diversion toilets have been resolutely rejected by the residents of informal settlements in Durban who want modern, flush toilets, just like the ones in middle-class homes. For them it is a modernist aspiration for human waste to be flushed away. Similarly, for the poo flingers in Cape Town, the new portable toilets are simply old buckets in new containers. They allow the smell of shit to waft through their shacks while they cook, eat, and sleep. They are also associated with everything about the apartheid past that the new democratic constitution claims to have overcome. By contrast, the porcelain flush toilet is a sign of modern citizenship in a democracy in which the disposal of human waste becomes the problem of state infrastructural systems; at the moment of flushing, shit then becomes matter out of sight and out of mind. This is the promise and expectation of democracy.

The iShack solar energy project, promoted by the Sustainability Institute in Stellenbosch, is meant to allow for incremental upgrades of 'slums' in South African cities. However, informal settlement residents in Enkanini rejected this project because they felt that solar power could not meet their energy needs (especially for large appliances such as fridges) and could jeopardize their demands on the local state for the provision of electrification, that is, 'proper power.'

Like TAC's rejection of claims that effective ART provision simply was not feasible in South Africa, the sanitation activist organizations SJC and Ses'khona have worked hard to increase the expectations of both communities and local governments and secure access to the 'global standards' of public health technology and infrastructure.

Conclusion

In this chapter, we sketched the outlines of a distinctive form of local resistance to global biomedical and public health intervention in South Africa. This resistance, however, does not take the form of a rejection of scientific forms of knowledge and practice and does not seek to assert the primacy of the local and the contextual over the global and universalizable. Rather, our examples, drawn from research with AIDS and sanitation activists, point to forms of political resistance that attempt to refigure the relationships between the political and the scientific, and the political and the global/local, in these interventions.

Activists here work to shift the political calculus of the usual invocations of scientific expertise and authority. They work against the typical ways in which the 'scientific' has been mystified and used to perpetuate conventional forms of development practice and health politics that exclude and deny. They also articulate a demand for access to a form of the global that is not diluted, compromised, or dumbed down for local consumption. This does not mean that they reject the importance of cultural and social differences, or are unaware of the practical constraints operating in their local contexts. They do, however, argue that discussions about 'the local' are often conducted and controlled by those who are not in fact local, and insist that gestures toward the local by external actors do not become ways of denying access to, or delivering inferior versions of, global technologies for health.

In doing so, these activists complicate the idea that global biomedical interventions necessarily deepen existing social and economic inequalities. To be sure, they articulate this politics in varying ways. Whereas SJC frames its interventions in terms of citizen rights to equal basic services and infrastructure, Ses'khona asserts its demands for equality in the language of a national liberation discourse derived from the anti-apartheid struggle. They seem to reject, at least implicitly, a Habermasian, deliberative democracy framing of human rights as the ground for claim-making (Dryzek, 2002). For Ses'khona, claims are rooted in reference to the notion of 'dignity,' an embodied, experiential, and affective claim that finds concrete, almost literal, expression in the poo protests. This is in stark contrast to the ways in which the TAC, SJC, and similar organizations (Equal Education, Ndifuna Ukwazi, and Section 27) use a combination of 'rights talk'/active citizenship, litigation, public pressure, and grassroots mobilization in order to persuade and lobby the state to meet its obligations to its citizens.

Whatever these differences in political perspective and strategy, however, all these organizations have found ways to challenge conventional styles of development and public health intervention effectively. Furthermore, in doing so, they have also found ways to avoid relying on romanticized forms of nativism and reflexive rejections of the 'modern' in favor of the 'traditional' when challenging these external actors and interventions. Recourses to these essentialized notions of the traditional and the local often have powerful, even 'strategic' (Spivak, 1988) logics of their own. We are not suggesting that these are irrational or illegitimate responses to global intervention, and indeed the other chapters in this volume have provided rich case studies of how these forms of resistance can be interpreted as meaningful and coherent responses to global intervention. We suggest, however, that the examples from the South African health activists described here provide valuable insight into another way in which local resistance to the global might be articulated and strategically deployed.

Editor commentary

Christopher Colvin and Steven Robins provide an intriguing comparison of organized resistance efforts. They show that resistance to global public health agendas

- Even when organized, can take on varied forms and political strategies, using combinations of active citizenship, litigation, public pressure, and grassroots mobilization.
- Strategically avoid the local or romanticized forms of nativism and reflexive rejection of scientific forms of knowledge and practice or the 'modern' in favor of the 'traditional'.
- Do not assert the primacy of the local and the contextual over the global and universal, while simultaneously not rejecting the impact of cultural and social differences and practical constraints in local contexts.
- Problematize discussions of the local by external actors.
- Challenge conventional styles of development and public health intervention that use science and expertise to exclude and deny.
- Reject the provision of inferior versions of global technologies for health.
- Refigure the relationships between the political and scientific, and the political and global/local, in public health policies and practices.

Notes

1 The African National Congress (ANC) is the dominant political party in South Africa, and has held power since the first democratic elections in 1994. The Western Cape Province,

however, voted in the Democratic Alliance party as their political representatives. These two primary political parties have conflicting views of many social and economic issues.

2 *Sunday Times*, 18 August 2013.

References

Ahmad, H. (2013). The Treatment Action Campaign and the three dimensions of lawyering: reflections from the rainbow nation. *SAHARA J*, *10*(1), 17-24. doi:10.1080/17290376.2013.807067

Appadurai, A. (2002). Deep democracy: Urban governmentality and the horizon of politics. *Public Culture*, *14*(1), 21–47.

Arendt, H. (1958). *The Human Condition*. Chicago: University of Chicago Press.

Biehl, J. (2007). Pharmaceuticalization: AIDS treatment and global health politics. *Anthropological Quarterly*, *80*(4), 1083-1126.

Colvin, C. J. (2012). True Believers or Modern Believers: HIV Science and the Work of the Dr Rath Foundation. In S. Levine (Ed.), *Medicine and the Politics of Knowledge* (pp. 33-54). Cape Town: Human Sciences Research Council.

Colvin, C. J., & Heywood, M. (2012). Negotiating ARV Prices with Pharmaceutical Companies and the South African Government: A Civil Sociey/Legal Approach. In E. Rosskam & I. Kikbusch (Eds.), *Negotiating and Navigating Global Health: Case Studies in Global Health Diplomacy*. London: Imperial College Press.

Colvin, C. J., & Robins, S. (2014). Social Movements after Apartheid: Rethinking Strategies and TACtics in a Time of Democratic Transition. In P. G. Klandermans & C. van Stralen (Eds.), *Movements in Times of Democratic Transition*: Temple University Press.

Dryzek, J. S. (2002). *Deliberative Democracy and Beyond: Liberals, Critics, Contestations*. Oxford: Oxford University Press.

Epstein, S. (1996). *Impure Science: AIDS, Activism, and the Politics of Knowledge*. Berkeley, CA: University of California Press.

Geffen, N. (2010). *Debunking Delusions: The Inside Story of the Treatment Action Campaign*. Auckland Park, South Africa: Jacana Media.

Herbert, B. (2001, June 11). In America; Refusing To Save Africans. *New York Times*. Retrieved from http://www.nytimes.com/2001/06/11/opinion/in-america-refusing-to-save-africans.html

Heywood, M. (2009). South Africa's Treatment Action Campaign: Combining law and social mobilization to realize the right to health. *Journal of Human Rights Practice*, *1*(1), 14-36.

Kalichman, S. (2009). *Denying AIDS: Conspiracy Theories, Pseudoscience, and Human Tragedy*. New York: Copernicus Books.

Kenyon, C. (2008). Cognitive dissonance as an explanation of the genesis, evolution and persistence of Thabo Mbeki's HIV denialism. *Afr J AIDS Res*, 7(1), 29-35. doi:10.2989/AJAR.2008.7.1.4.432

Kielmann, K., & Cataldo, F. (2010). Tracking the rise of the "expert patient" in evolving paradigms of HIV care. *AIDS Care*, *22 Suppl 1*, 21-28. doi:10.1080/09540121003721000

Laporte, D. (2000). *The History of Shit*. Cambridge, MA: MIT Press.

Lewis, J. (Writer). (2011). *TAC: Taking HAART*. In L. B. Jack Lewis (Producer): Community Media Trust.

Lievrouw, L. A. (2011). *Alternative and Activist New Media*. Cambridge, UK ; Malden, MA: Polity.

Mbali, M. (2013). *South African AIDS Activism and Global Health Politics*. Houndmills, Basingstoke, Hampshire: Palgrave Macmillan.

Mehta, L., & Movik, S. (2011). *Shit Matters: The Potential of Community-Led Total Sanitation.* Warwickshire, UK: Practical Action Publishing.

Nattrass, N. (2004). *The Moral Economy of AIDS in South Africa.* Cambridge: Cambridge University Press.

Nattrass, N. (2007). *Mortal Combat: AIDS Denialism and the Struggle for Antiretrovirals in South Africa.* Scottsville, South Africa: University of KwaZulu-Natal Press.

Nattrass, N. (2010). Still crazy after all these years: The challenge of AIDS denialism for science. *AIDS Behav, 14*(2), 248-251. doi:10.1007/s10461-009-9641-z

Nattrass, N. (2012). *The AIDS conspiracy : science fights back.* New York: Columbia University Press.

Nixon, R. (2011). *Slow Violence and the Environmentalism of the Poor.* Cambridge, MA.: Harvard University Press.

Rasnik, D. (2005). Talk with President Mbeki. Retrieved from http://www.virusmyth.net/aids/news/drtalkmbeki.htm

Robins, S. (2009). Foot soldiers of global health: Teaching and preaching AIDS science and modern medicine on the frontline. *Medical Anthropology, 28*(1), 81-107.

Robins, S. (2014a). The 2011 toilet wars in South Africa: Justice and transition between the exceptional and the everyday after apartheid. *Development and Change, 45*(3), 479-501.

Robins, S. (2014b). Poo wars as matter out of place: 'Toilets for Africa' in Cape Town. *Anthropology Today, 30*(1), 1-3.

Robins, S. (2014c). Slow activism in fast times: Reflections on the politics of media spectacles after apartheid. *Journal of Southern African Studies, 40*(1), 91-110.

Smith, R. A., & Siplon, P. D. (2006). *Drugs into Bodies: Global AIDS Treatment Activism.* Westport, CT: Praeger.

Social Justice Coalition. (2010). Memorandum on the results of the water sampling in RR Section, conducted by Dr. J.M. Barnes, Division of Community Health. Cape Town: Social Justice Coalition.

Social Justice Coalition. (2013). Report of the Khayelitsha 'Mshengu' Toilet Social Audit. Cape Town: Social Justice Coalition.

Spivak, G. (1988). Can the Subaltern Speak? In C. Nelson & L. Grossberg (Eds.), *Marxism and the Interpretation of Culture* (pp. 271-313). Basingstoke: Macmillan Education.

Stinson, K., Giddy, J., Cox, V., Burton, R., Ibeto, M., Cragg, C.,...Goemaere, E. (2014). Reflections on a decade of delivering PMTCT in Khayelitsha, South Africa. *Southern African Journal of HIV Medicine, 15*(1), 30-32.

Yamin, A. E., & Gloppen, S. (2011). *Litigating Health Rights: Can Courts Bring More Justice to Health?* Cambridge, MA: Human Rights Program Harvard University Press.

INDEX